# An Amazing Little Girl with Rhombencephalosynapsis

Stephanie Detjen Costabel

Copyright: 2022

No part of this book may be reproduced in any form or by any electronic or mechanical means, or the facilitation thereof, including information storage and retrieval systems, without permission in writing from the publisher, except in the case of brief quotations published in articles and reviews. Any educational institution wishing to photocopy part or all of the work for classroom use, or individual researchers who would like to obtain permission to reprint the work for educational purposes, should contact the publisher

ISBN: 978-0-578-36087-4.

Cover and interior design by Diana Wade

Editor: Betsy Thorpe

Copy Editor: Kathy Brown

Cover photograph by Sarah Nelson Conklin Photography

Printed in the United States of America

stephanie.costabel@hotmail.com

# CONTENTS

Prologue . . . . . . . . . . . . . . . . . . . . . . . . . . . . . . . . . . . . . . . . . . . 1
1. . . . . . . . . . . . . . . . . . . . . . . . . . . . . . . . . . . . . . . . . . . . . . . . . 3
2. . . . . . . . . . . . . . . . . . . . . . . . . . . . . . . . . . . . . . . . . . . . . . . . . 9
3. . . . . . . . . . . . . . . . . . . . . . . . . . . . . . . . . . . . . . . . . . . . . . . 15
4. . . . . . . . . . . . . . . . . . . . . . . . . . . . . . . . . . . . . . . . . . . . . . . 25
5. . . . . . . . . . . . . . . . . . . . . . . . . . . . . . . . . . . . . . . . . . . . . . . 33
6. . . . . . . . . . . . . . . . . . . . . . . . . . . . . . . . . . . . . . . . . . . . . . . 41
7. . . . . . . . . . . . . . . . . . . . . . . . . . . . . . . . . . . . . . . . . . . . . . . 51
8. . . . . . . . . . . . . . . . . . . . . . . . . . . . . . . . . . . . . . . . . . . . . . . 61
9. . . . . . . . . . . . . . . . . . . . . . . . . . . . . . . . . . . . . . . . . . . . . . . 71
10. . . . . . . . . . . . . . . . . . . . . . . . . . . . . . . . . . . . . . . . . . . . . . 81
11. . . . . . . . . . . . . . . . . . . . . . . . . . . . . . . . . . . . . . . . . . . . . . 91
12. . . . . . . . . . . . . . . . . . . . . . . . . . . . . . . . . . . . . . . . . . . . . . 99
13. . . . . . . . . . . . . . . . . . . . . . . . . . . . . . . . . . . . . . . . . . . . . 107
14. . . . . . . . . . . . . . . . . . . . . . . . . . . . . . . . . . . . . . . . . . . . . 117
15. . . . . . . . . . . . . . . . . . . . . . . . . . . . . . . . . . . . . . . . . . . . . 125
16. . . . . . . . . . . . . . . . . . . . . . . . . . . . . . . . . . . . . . . . . . . . . 131
17. . . . . . . . . . . . . . . . . . . . . . . . . . . . . . . . . . . . . . . . . . . . . 141
18. . . . . . . . . . . . . . . . . . . . . . . . . . . . . . . . . . . . . . . . . . . . . 151
19. . . . . . . . . . . . . . . . . . . . . . . . . . . . . . . . . . . . . . . . . . . . . 161
20. . . . . . . . . . . . . . . . . . . . . . . . . . . . . . . . . . . . . . . . . . . . . 165
21. . . . . . . . . . . . . . . . . . . . . . . . . . . . . . . . . . . . . . . . . . . . . 171
22. . . . . . . . . . . . . . . . . . . . . . . . . . . . . . . . . . . . . . . . . . . . . 183
23. . . . . . . . . . . . . . . . . . . . . . . . . . . . . . . . . . . . . . . . . . . . . 193
24. . . . . . . . . . . . . . . . . . . . . . . . . . . . . . . . . . . . . . . . . . . . . 201
25. . . . . . . . . . . . . . . . . . . . . . . . . . . . . . . . . . . . . . . . . . . . . 211
26. . . . . . . . . . . . . . . . . . . . . . . . . . . . . . . . . . . . . . . . . . . . . 217
27. . . . . . . . . . . . . . . . . . . . . . . . . . . . . . . . . . . . . . . . . . . . . 221

# Acknowledgments

To the doctors, nurses, therapists, teachers, and specialists working with Alessia: Thank you for all you have done to help my girl. Without your dedication and patience, Alessia wouldn't have come so far.

To my mother and sisters, thank you for always being there for me. Always lending me a helping hand, encouraging me through tough times. You have had my back from day one and I will forever cherish your love.

To Mika, thank you for believing in my Alessia. You have been my go-to person, my right hand, my advocate. Your devotion in helping children with special needs is incredible. I hope you know how amazing you are.

To Dr. Jennifer Squires, to your dedication to medicine. You are a gift in Alessia's life. Your constant research and determination to help my Alessia. I am so thankful to have chosen you as my children's pediatrician.

To the Rhomebencephalosynapsis support Facebook group. Thanking all of you for your incredible knowledge, advice, and hope.

To my husband, for the sleepless nights of endless worry we shared. You have been my shoulder to cry on. We have gone through this journey together, as a team, as soulmates. I love you more than you will ever know.

To my children, Thiago and Sophia. Thank you for your understanding, for being my rock. For putting up with my bad mood in the hardest times. You two give me the strength to keep going. Thank you for loving me and your sister unconditionally. Don't ever underestimate your self-worth, intelligence, and uniqueness. You two are extraordinary human beings and Mama is immensely proud of you.

The completion of this book could have not been possible without the participation and assistance of my editor, Betsy Thorpe, copy editor Kathy Brown, and my graphic designer, Diane Wade. Thank you for your guidance and support in bringing this memoir to life.

# An Amazing Little Girl with Rhombencephalosynapsis

*"Even though our journey as parents of a medically fragile child began with emotional turmoil, it has since become a purposeful odyssey that brings meaning and depth to our lives. This is the road we were born to travel."*
—Charisse Montgomery

*"I have slept in a hospital chair, skipped meals, cried from fear and joy. I have become an expert on my child's condition. I am a strong advocate and have had to make life changing decisions. I am the parent of a medically complex warrior."*
—Unknown

*"Sometimes, real superheroes live in the hearts of small children fighting big battles."*
—Unknown

*"We are not only parents; we become nurses, therapists, chauffeurs, companions and more . . . For some of us the needs of our child are so time-consuming that working outside of the home becomes impossible and impractical."*
—Silvia Corpadin

*"There comes a point where it all becomes too much. When we get too tired to fight anymore so we give up. That's when the real work begins . . . to find hope where there seems to be absolutely none at all."*
—Cristina Yang

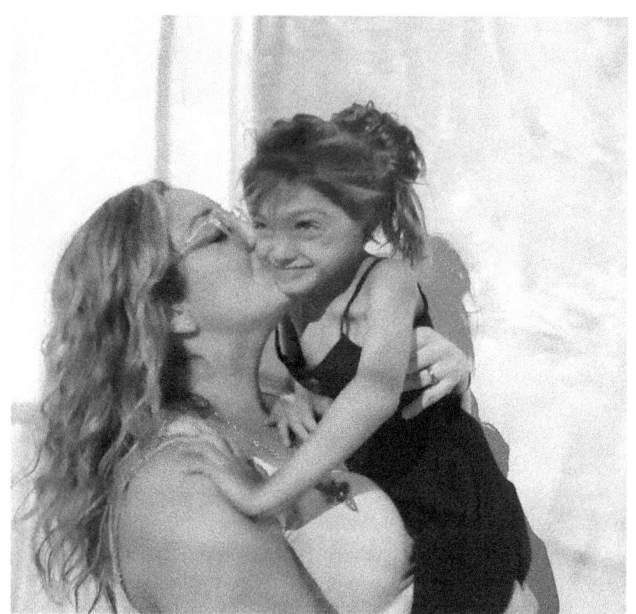

*Alessia and me, 2021. Photo Credit: Ronaldo Cruz*

# An Amazing Little Girl with Rhombencephalosynapsis

My Dearest Alessia,

There is nothing I wouldn't do for you. From the moment I saw your beautiful little face, I immediately fell in love. You have been the light of my eyes. You have taught me in these last six years more than I have ever learned in my entire life.

You have taught me to understand how fragile and delicate life truly is. You have taught me to see and enjoy every single minute of life that I see your smiling face and that of your siblings. You have taught me to appreciate and not take for granted those little moments the rest of the world takes for granted.

The gift of being able to swallow and taste my morning coffee. The gift of not living in constant pain. The gift of seeing the beauty of nature. Those vivid green colors of the trees and the grass. The gift of hearing the beautiful tunes of music or the birds chirping and singing at sunrise. The gift of breathing. There is nothing more valuable than being alive and healthy.

You have taught me what it means to be persistent. You have taught me the true value of patience. You have taught me that anyone can adapt to their current life situations. That there is nothing stronger than the will to live. I would change every single medical battle you have had to face, but I would never in a million years change your personality. You are fierce. You are determined. You have the strength of a warrior. You are the bravest, strongest person I have ever had the pleasure of meeting. This is your story. This is your legacy.

The love I have for you and your siblings is the strongest love I have ever known. And I will never stop advocating for you. You are a gift to this world and there is so much to learn from you. I hope one day you will truly understand the immense impact you have had on the lives of everyone that knows you. I love you beyond measure and I hope one day you will understand how incredibly amazing you are.

With Much Love,
Mama

# Prologue

Parenting a special-needs child with complex medical needs changes you in a way you would never think possible. You can't truly grasp what it is like, until you live it. The first few years will pull you so far away from who you were that you won't even recognize yourself. You will find yourself looking at the mirror and wondering whatever happened to the "you" you used to be. You will find yourself in a crowded room and feel isolated and alone, thinking about why this happened to you . . . why it did not happen to someone else . . . why your child and not theirs?

It will challenge your marriage, your relationships with your friends and your family. You will want to scream at the top of your lungs why nobody can understand your frustration, your depression, or your constant irritability.

It will challenge your relationship with God. You will question your faith. You will question just about everything you used to believe. You will envy everyone that has healthy children.

The children's hospital will be your second home. You will see your doctors, nurses, and therapists more than your friends or family. You will argue with them. You will look for second, third, and even fourth opinions, trying to escape reality with the hopes one of them will tell you what you want to hear. You will think doctors are looking at you like you are paranoid. They are used to this. We—new mothers to sick kids—clearly are not. You will hold your screaming child down while the nurses insert not one, but two, or three IVs. You will hate it and wish you were the one getting poked and not your child. You will cry. God, you will cry so much.

Often, people will say things to you that will irritate you. "God only gives you what you can handle." "You are so strong; I wouldn't be able to do it." "Pray more and she will get better." "You just haven't been praying hard enough." "She came to teach us a lesson." And so many other comments that will boil your blood.

The truth is that you are strong because being strong is the only option you have. I choose to believe God has nothing to do with it. It took me years to believe that. But everyone comes to a different belief, and it's okay! People say things because they don't know what else to say. If they were in your shoes, certainly, they would think differently.

This is the story of an amazing little girl with Rhombencephalosynapsis. My daughter. Alessia. I am sharing her story the way our family lived it. What we went through. What we learned. I am her voice since she has none. She is an incredible human being that has gone through more in six years than most of us adults go through in a lifetime. My hope is that you gain a better understanding of what it means to be a special-needs family and how you can use her story as inspiration to fully understand how precious, delicate, and valuable life truly is.

If you are new to the special needs/medically complex journey, I want you to know that you are not alone. Medically complex children live an unimaginably difficult life. You wonder how you can find happiness while you see your child in so much pain. You live in fight-or-flight mode 24/7. But through it all, you learn so much. You learn things you would have never learned had you not had your child. Happiness is truly possible, even in the worst scenarios. You learn to see life differently . . . to understand entirely the meaning of appreciating and enjoying the small things.

# 1

I was thirteen weeks pregnant with my second baby. I was going to see my baby for the first time at my first ultrasound appointment. The clinic had scheduled me for late in the afternoon—I didn't get off work until 5 p.m. I went alone to the appointment, because my husband, Ronaldo, had to go pick up our three-year-old son, Thiago, at daycare. On that cold December day, the rain was pouring on my windshield as I was driving towards the clinic, and the skies were dark. It was hard to see through the foggy windows.

I was the last patient, so the only people at the clinic were the ultrasound technician and myself. I walked into the clinic feeling comfortable and relaxed. Honestly, I just wanted to make sure the baby was where it needed to be and had a strong heartbeat.

The ultrasound technician walked me to the room. She gave me a blanket and said she would be right back. I was shaking while I tried to warm up underneath the blanket because of the cold in that room. The technician applied the ultrasound gel on my belly and started the procedure. To add to my chill, the gel was freezing. I wasn't even looking at the screen until I heard the technician give a little a chuckle, and say, "Oh wow . . . there's two in there."

"Two what?" I asked.

I looked at the screen and sure enough, I saw two little babies, side-by-side. I couldn't believe my eyes. I was in shock—surprised and worried all at the same time. "Are you sure?" I asked. "How is that even possible? I have no twins in the family. Oh my God, how the hell am I going to do this? It's going to be so much work!"

"Yeah, it is a lot of work," she replied as she smiled at the two distinct bodies on the monitor. I looked at the image on the monitor. Ronaldo was not going to be happy.

It had taken me a whole year to convince him to have another baby. He already had a 10-year-old daughter from a previous relationship, and our son. Ronaldo's daughter lived in Nicaragua and only came to visit us on summer breaks. But I'd felt like Thiago needed a sibling that lived with us. I had always wanted two children back-to-back so they wouldn't have a big age difference. We argued constantly about the issue, to the point of considering divorce. Finally, Ronaldo agreed to have another baby.

I noticed the technician's expression change. Her eyebrows furrowed and her smile turned into a frown. She had seen something on the monitor that was concerning. What was it? I looked at her trying to decipher what she had seen on the monitor. She quickly excused herself from the room and told me she was going to call the doctor and would be right back. I nervously picked up my phone and called Ronaldo. As soon as he picked up, I started crying. I was so nervous and the only words that I was able to say were, "Oh my God, I am so sorry, there are two. Oh my God, we are having twins!" There was a long pause. He too was in shock, but also sounded excited and happy. We were both speechless. I told him to go to my mom's house with Thiago and I would meet him there once the technician returned and finished the procedure.

After what seemed to be about an hour, the technician finally returned. Her expression was different, peculiar. "I need to take some more pictures," she said.

think it happens to other people, not you. Then this miraculous child comes into your life, and everything changes. But you learn. You see life differently. You see beautiful things most people don't have the opportunity to see.

It took years for me to understand this.

Sitting in my car that day, I had no idea the person I would become. I had no idea the little person growing in my belly would be a true miracle. An angel on Earth.

And so, the start of this amazing journey began that cold, rainy, seventeenth day of December.

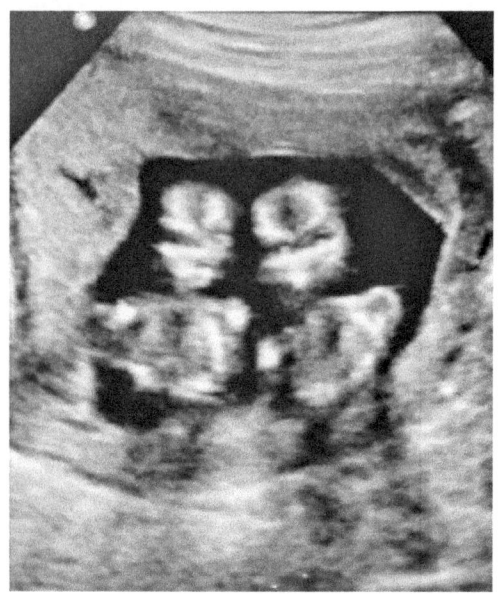

*First picture of my girls, December 2014*
*Photo Credit: Caromont Imaging Services*

# 2

I graduated from the University of North Carolina at Charlotte with a major in International Studies, concentrating on Latin America. My dream job was to work at an embassy in foreign affairs. I did not know at the time how incredibly difficult it was to find a job in that field of study. I never had any luck finding my dream job, so I settled in working at an office for a property management firm. While I was there, I started gaining interest in the real estate business. I went to real estate school to prepare for the North Carolina Real Estate exam to get licensed.

I had a normal life back then. I had a simple nine-to-five job. Ronaldo was starting his window-tinting business and Thiago was going to daycare. I figured that if I could get into real estate, I would have more flexibility in my work schedule and be able to care for my second baby that I wished to have the following year.

I found out about my MoMo twins a week before I took my NC Real Estate exam. I studied night and day for that exam and was confident I was going to pass. But it's amazing how your brain can get fixated in a constant state of worry. No matter how many times I would read each question on that exam, I just could NOT concentrate. My mind was on my MoMo twin pregnancy.

I knew I was going to have to quit my job since I had to be admitted at twenty-four weeks. I joined a group on Facebook formed to support new mothers in their MoMo pregnancy journey. It was formed by a deeply knowledgeable group of mothers that had first-hand experience. There was excellent advice on how to deal with the emotional strain and anxiety of your pregnancy, as well as tips for when you were admitted. There were also many mothers who had lost one or both of their babies. Some even lost their babies at thirty-two weeks. The group recommended not having a baby shower until your babies made it to twenty-four weeks, since so many pregnancies were lost.

So, obviously I worried. A lot. Constantly.

I ended up failing the NC State Real Estate exam twice that month. I decided I was just going to get back to real estate once I had my twins. I've learned that when you are juggling too many balls at once, you must let one drop, for your own sanity. So real estate was just going to have to wait.

I had a lot of planning to do. I had met with a perinatalogist that put a date, March 9, 2015, when I was going to be admitted to closely monitor the pregnancy. I had two and a half months to prepare for my absence at work and at home.

January 12, 2015: My mother, Ronaldo, and I were super excited. We were going to find out the sex of the twins! We dropped Thiago off at daycare and went straight to the appointment. We joked that if they were boys, Ronaldo was going to have a full window-tinting crew for his business. I wanted girls, since I already had a son, but was still content with whatever sex they were. Honestly, I just wanted to be able to meet them. My mind kept on bringing up the fear that I wouldn't even make it to twenty-four weeks.

We arrived at the clinic, checked in, and waited to be called. Nervous, we found it hard to wait. We were so eager to know. They finally called me and all three of us went back. The technician started the ultrasound and we waited patiently. We could not remove our eyeballs from the monitor. But one baby was on top of the other, and the sexes couldn't be determined. I moved around trying to get one of the babies to move.

Suddenly, they moved! Their distinct bodies were now completely visible on the monitor. Girls! We were going to have twin girls.

My mind flooded with pink. Two sweet, pink bundles of joy. I thought to myself, "They are going to be mini-me's." My mom and Ronaldo broke into huge smiles. I was so incredibly happy in that moment. Soon after, worry overpowered me again. What if they died? What if I didn't make it to twenty-four weeks?

After the appointment, we went to IHOP for brunch to celebrate the fact I was having girls. We made jokes on how Ronaldo and Thiago were the only boys in the family. We were fantasizing on how beautiful the girls would be with my eyes and his hair. We even were joking on how they would be mischievous and make us grow grey hairs when they were teenagers.

I couldn't stop worrying, though. All I could think of in that IHOP was, "Please, God, let them survive."

The following two and a half months I prayed.

I have never been a deeply religious person. My religious beliefs at the time were that an energy, a force, a higher being called God existed, offered guidance, and answered prayers. So, I prayed.

Prayer gives you hope. The hope that your prayers will be answered. The feeling that God has control on any difficult situation, and that he will always protect you. And so, I prayed daily.

I prayed my girls would make it to twenty-four weeks. I prayed and begged God to make sure they wouldn't die. I prayed they would both be completely healthy and normal. I prayed Thiago would not resent me for not being home for two months. I lived with that heavy worry on my shoulders that I could not control. My time of release was every night in the shower. Every night I would let the water run down my cheeks and I cried. I would pray, "Please, God, don't allow us to have a child with any medical problems. If your plan is for one of my daughters to die or to have disabilities, please just take them both now." I was scared to have a child with disabilities.

People don't understand special needs or disabilities until they are directly affected by a family member with disabilities. You see them occasionally, at a mall, or at a restaurant . . . you might stare or be intrigued, but then you just shrug. You understand that they are not "normal" and might feel sorry for them and their families. I thought like that at the time, but oh, how I was mistaken.

I managed to rely on my faith and was able to convince myself that everything was going to be okay. That I was going to have beautiful, perfect, healthy twin girls.

At work, everyone was preparing for my absence. I was going to be out for two months while inpatient, and three months afterwards for maternity leave. My position was important, and the company could not just put my job on hold, so they found someone else to do the job and I spent my last month training this person. They prepared a baby shower for me before I left. The company was extremely happy with me and appreciative of my work. I knew I was going to be missed.

My last day at work was March 6. It was a bittersweet day. I had to say goodbye to some amazing coworkers and pack up my stuff.

The human mind is designed to maintain its emotional stability when it knows what to expect. But I had no idea what to expect at the time. I was not going to have an income. I did not know at the time that I could have applied for disability. I was going to rely solely on Ronaldo for finances. I did not like that idea. I have always been an independent woman. The thought of not working or having an income freaked me out a little.

My only hope was that it was going to be temporary. It was just going to be a break, that's all. I would be back in the workforce in no time. Just a few months . . . only those months ended up being years. Oh, how did my plan go awry.

Every day that went by was a mini victory. I would say to myself, I am one day closer. Suddenly, the day arrived. I had made it to twenty-four weeks.

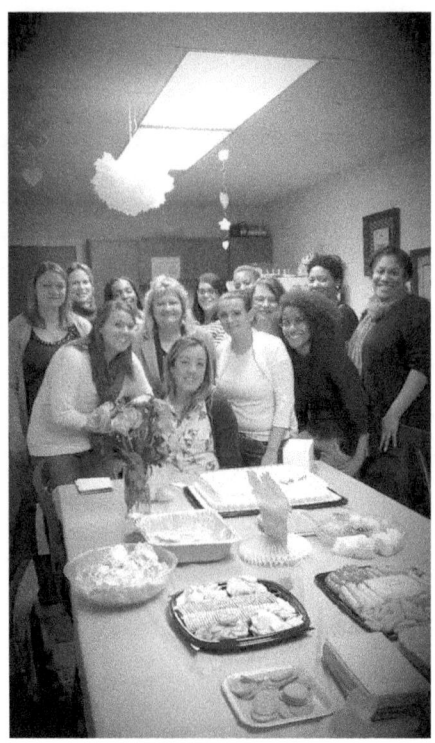

*My baby shower at work, January 2015*
*Photo Credit: Ben Kincel*

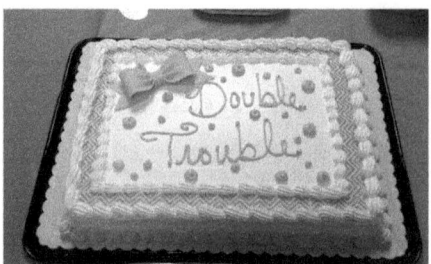

*My baby shower cake, January 2015*
*Photo Credit: Stephanie Detjen Costabel*

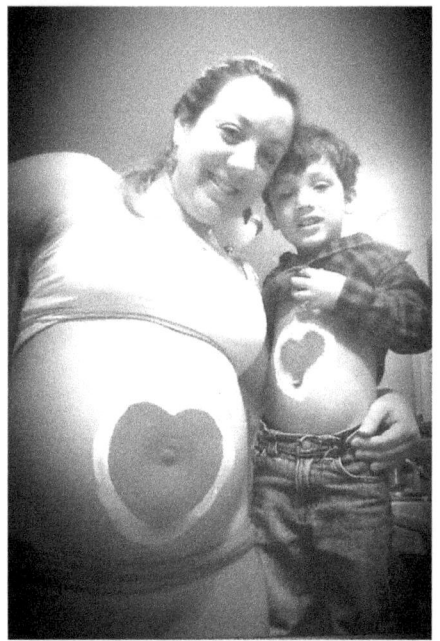

*Thiago and me, at 20 weeks pregnant with the girls, February 2015.*
*Photo Credit: Stephanie Detjen Costabel*

# 3

The night before I was admitted to the hospital, I made sure to pack anything that was going to make my hospital room feel like home. My pillow, bed comforter, nightlight, towels, pictures of Thiago. I had five huge bags of stuff. It seemed like I was moving to the hospital.

I had prepared myself psychologically. If I could keep myself entertained during those eight weeks, it wasn't going to be that bad, I reasoned. I took my acrylic paints and paintbrushes, along with ten blank canvases. My goal was to paint all day, every day. I've always liked to paint abstract art of my feelings or images I have in my head. There is something about painting that brings tranquility to the soul. I like the feeling of accomplishment when I see my finished artwork, especially if it turns out well.

March 9 started liked any other day. My mother, Ronaldo, and I stopped to drop Thiago off at daycare before heading to Carolinas Medical Center Main Hospital. Thiago did not understand at the time that Mommy wasn't going to be home for a while. He would be able to visit me at the hospital, but I would not be at home. As I said goodbye to him, I couldn't contain my tears. It seemed like two months was going to be an eternity. I left the daycare as quickly as possible. I felt like I was going to cry a river if I stayed more than I had to.

We arrived at the hospital and checked in. Eighth floor, the

Antepartum Unit. To get to that unit you had to cross the normal Labor and Delivery unit where all the normal pregnancies went. I would pass the rooms and see family members hanging around outside the rooms. New moms carrying their babies. It was a bittersweet feeling. I wished I were having a normal pregnancy like that. It seemed so easy compared to my situation.

I was given the biggest room in the antepartum unit. They save these rooms for mothers that must be inpatient for a long time. I settled in and appreciated the large windows that dominated the whole wall in front of my hospital bed. I could see the main entrance of the hospital, the greenway, as well as the outdoor fresh market where they sold plants and organic vegetables. It was spectacular.

I was settling into my room smoothly, until the nurse came in and said they had to place an IV in my arm. That's when I lost it. I thought I was going to be monitored three times a day until the babies reached thirty-two weeks. "But why on Earth would I need an IV for two months?" I asked.

The nurse explained that an IV must be placed in case they had to do an emergency C-section if the babies suddenly became distressed. I was terrified of needles. I demanded to talk to the resident OB-GYN because I was NOT going to have an IV in my vein for two months, "just in case."

The OB-GYN walked into the room. She was probably in her mid-thirties. She sat next to me at the bedside. "Mrs. Costabel, you do understand that your babies can die if we have to have an emergency C-section while you are here and they can't stick an IV into you, right?" I furrowed my eyebrows and looked straight into her eyes.

"My veins are plump. I am sure we can wait a few weeks to put an IV in. I am an excellent stick." She nodded and agreed to wait a few weeks for the IV placement. It was a relief. Looking back, the IV wasn't the worst part of my hospital stay. It was just the start.

The way they would monitor the babies was to attach a belt on my belly with two heart monitors. One for Twin A and the other for Twin B. Those were the names of my babies at the hospital. It would always take the nurses a while to find the heartbeats of the babies, so I would have to stay still while they searched. I had to have this monitoring four times a day for one hour each time. If there was a dip in either of the babies' heartrates, known as a desaturation, they would add another hour of monitoring. The babies had to have a full hour without desaturations before I was able to have the belt removed and could walk around again.

Some days went by uneventfully. Some days, I was stuck lying on my hospital bed for hours, because just when the hour of monitoring was almost up, one of the babies would have a desaturation and an extra hour of monitoring was added.

This grew old very fast. I am not the type of person who can just lie for hours in a bed. Especially since I felt totally fine. I needed to walk around my room, go to the cafeteria, take a breath of fresh air outside. It's amazing how these simple things become so important to you when you can't do them.

I started getting depressed.

Ronaldo and Thiago would come to the hospital to have dinner with me every evening from 6 p.m. to 9 p.m. I would use this time to do crafts with Thiago or watch a movie. He loved seeing me. I cried every single time they left, because Thiago never wanted to leave and always left with a sad expression. My poor boy.

My mother, sisters, and some friends would come on the weekends to visit me. But visits would only be a few hours and then I would be all alone. I hated the loneliness I felt during that time. I wanted to make it to thirty-two weeks so badly, but the days were incredibly long. When I wasn't on the monitor, I painted my canvases. It was a way to distract my brain from the loneliness and for the days to go by faster. I painted a lion and a giraffe for Thiago, baby girl owls on a tree branch for my twins, an abstract guitar for Ronaldo, a colorful tree for my mom, and another abstract tree for my house. By the time my inpatient stay at the hospital was over, my whole room looked like an art gallery.

The nurses taking care of me became my friends. To this day, I am still in touch with some of them. For Easter, I helped one of the nurses paint little flowerpots for the antepartum rooms. I had an Easter Egg hunt with Thiago in my hospital room. He would always ask when I was coming home.

After six weeks in the hospital, thirty weeks into my pregnancy, I started having complications. The twins were much bigger and the space in my womb was getting tight. The umbilical cords were getting dangerously tangled. Their heartrates were now being monitored continuously because they were having many desaturations. I had to lie on that hospital bed with the monitor belt on 24/7. My back was killing me. I was so ready for them to be born.

The day arrived when it was just too dangerous for them to stay inside of me any longer. The umbilical cords were tight and tangled, and oxygen was decreasing to the babies.

April 15, 2015, at 10 a.m., my twin girls were born via C-section at thirty weeks' gestation.

I had waited for six weeks in the hospital to finally meet them, and I was so nervous. It seemed surreal that I was finally going to see them. I had made it. I was going to have two live babies. They had made it. They had survived. I was so incredibly relieved.

As soon as the doctor took my babies out of my womb, they were immediately rushed to the NICU. They were ten weeks premature, so they needed help breathing. I kept asking Ronaldo if he could see them. He was pale. He had a good glimpse of all my insides. "They are here, baby." He smiled as he caressed my forehead. I was able to see Sophia's face briefly. She had been Twin A. The first one out. I didn't get a chance to see Alessia's face. The doctors rushed her to the NICU. I would have to wait till after I was out of recovery to be able to see Alessia. It would be nighttime by then.

The NICU can be heaven for some parents, but it can also be hell. Babies are lost in the NICU, but also miracles happen. When you walk in, you see tiny babies in incubators. Most have breathing tubes, CPAPs, monitors, IVs, and machines alarming constantly. It can be a scary place.

That night, I was wheelchaired into the NICU to see my girls. I wasn't sure at the time what exactly I was expecting to see. They were ten weeks premature, so obviously they were going to have millions of tubes all over their small bodies. They were situated at opposite ends of the NICU. I went to see Sophia first. It was really hard to see your newborn daughter with an IV on her head and so many tubes coming out of her tiny little body. You have a baby, and you picture it with perfect rosy cheeks. Healthy for sure. When you have a premature baby, it's totally different. I was shocked at how my baby was fighting for her life. She looked so helpless, struggling so hard to breathe. The machines alarmed constantly. It knocked the wind out of me.

Before I could truly grasp what I was seeing, the NICU doctor approached me and said, "Hi, Mrs. Costabel. Congratulations on your twins. Hey, there is something I need to show you about Twin B." Twin B was Alessia. Why on Earth could the doctor just not have used her real name?

I was quickly led to my other baby, Alessia. She looked just like Sophia, with tubes all over the place and an IV on her head. The NICU doctor showed me her left ear. To my surprise it was missing. It looked like a tiny little peanut of cartilage but there was no ear canal or hole. It was completely closed. The NICU doctor said they hadn't noticed it when she was born. They just noticed it when Alessia got down to the NICU. She said it was called microtia and was just a birth defect.

Mothers know when something is not right. I wasn't worried about her not having an ear and how she would look physically. I worried that there could be something deeper, and whether she would be deaf in that ear. I wondered if there was something else wrong with her. I mentioned it to the doctor, and she agreed on having genetic testing done. That night I cried, because I had a feeling there was something else more than just her ear missing. Something was terribly wrong.

I went back to my hospital room and tried to sleep. I was worried about Alessia. Anxiety took over, like I was emotionally preparing myself for an unexpected piece of information that would be devastating. I tried to just block these thoughts out of my head and go to sleep. I prayed hard that night. I fell asleep thinking to myself, it will be okay, it's just a birth defect, everything will be fine.

I was incredibly mistaken. But at the time I lived with false hope, and that's how I managed my anxiety.

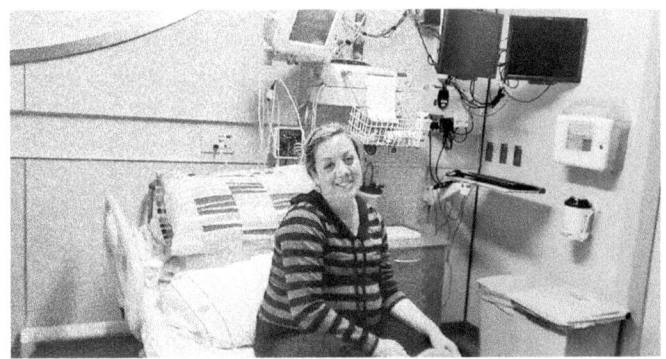

*First day of my inpatient stay, March 2015*
*Photo Credit: Cristina Costabel*

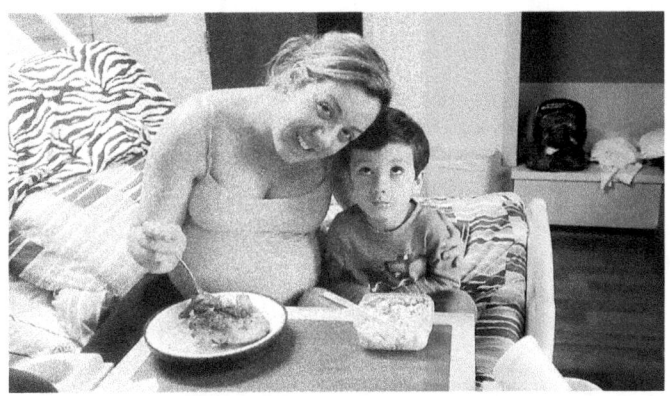

*Thiago visiting me at the hospital, March 2015*
*Photo Credit: Cristina Costabel*

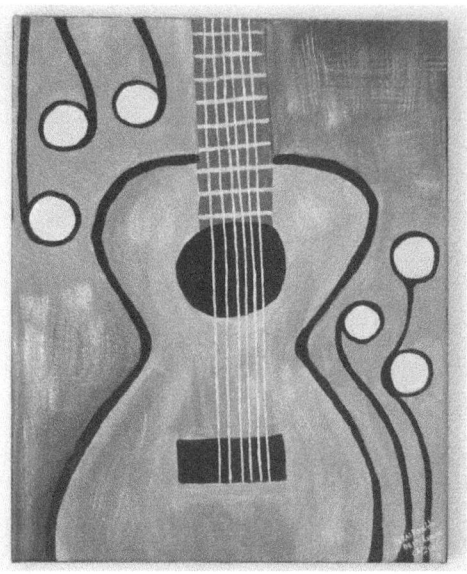

*Some of my artwork from my inpatient stay, March 2015*
*All Photos Credit: Stephanie Detjen Costabel*

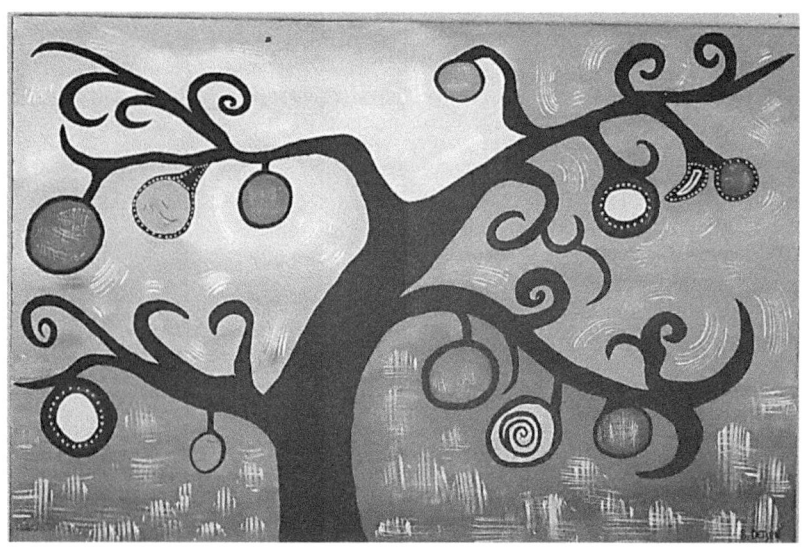

## An Amazing Little Girl with Rhombencephalosynapsis

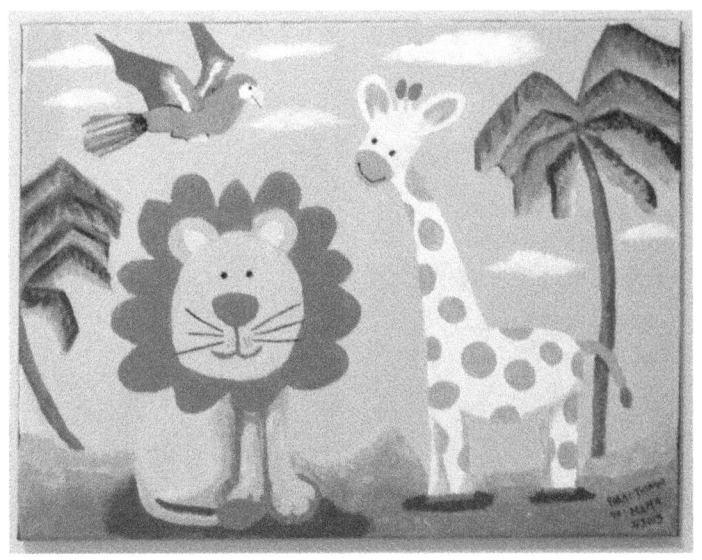

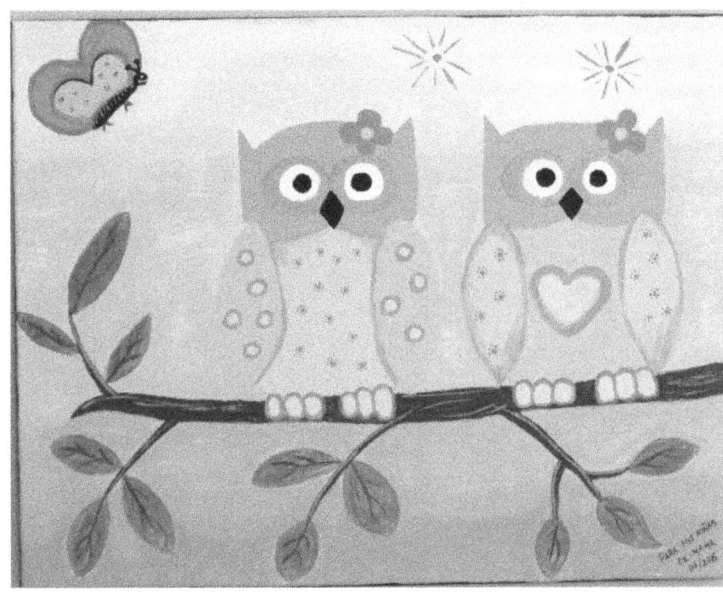

# 4

Most women dream about the day they become mothers. Their nine-month pregnancy is filled with excitement and planning for the new baby. They decorate the nursery, have a baby shower, and deliver a healthy full-term baby. After about two or three days they are discharged from the hospital with their newborn. They go home with the new member of the family, a bundle of joy.

When you have a premature baby, or babies in my case, that fantasyland turns into a world of chaos. The sounds of the alarms of the multiple machines in the NICU, the constant doctor and nurse calls to check on your baby, machines pumping milk out of your breasts because your baby is too premature to breastfeed. Your breast milk is put into a syringe connected to a feeding tube. NICU nurses have to place a feeding tube down your baby's nose or throat to give them their nutrition, because your baby can't coordinate its swallowing and breathing all at the same time.

There are so many emotions, adrenaline, and excitement of meeting your baby, then sadness of seeing your baby struggling to breathe with multiple IVs on their fragile, little body. The anger that they are so sick. The guilt you couldn't keep them in your belly longer. The envy you feel when you see new mothers carrying their newborns out of the hospital doors while they wait for their husbands to get the car. The fear every time you hear the alarms of the monitors going off alerting the nurses a baby forgot to breathe.

Three days after my C-section, it was finally time for me to go home. I had looked forward to this moment for so long that I had not thought about how I was going to feel going home without my girls.

I felt so helpless leaving them, but I had no choice. They needed time to grow. I was sore and in pain from my C-section. My breasts were sore from pumping. I kept telling myself, "Hey, at least they both survived, right?" So many mothers lose their babies to this type of pregnancy that I was grateful to have two live babies. But at the same time, I couldn't stop worrying about Alessia and her missing ear.

When Thiago saw me come home, I found tremendous support and happiness just seeing how excited and happy Thiago was. His little face was lit up like a little boy on his birthday. I was also relieved to be back home. Sleeping in my bed, with no interruptions from nurses, no noises, and the company of my husband was beautiful. But I thought a lot about my girls. I kept telling myself, "They'll be home soon, and the hospital will just be a distant memory."

I didn't get to hold my babies until twelve days after they were born. They had been intubated for the first couple of days, and after the breathing tube came out, they were still on a high flow CPAP machine and too fragile to be held. Finally, at twelve days old, my babies were stable enough to hold them up against my chest. In the NICU, this is called "skin-to-skin contact" and is supposed to help with the growth of premature babies. This was the way they needed to be held.

For this to happen, the nurses must make sure that the baby's heart rate, respiratory, and oxygen monitors maintain connectivity with the machines. All the cables must be carefully secured to one side while they take the baby out of the incubator. The IV lines also must be carefully held, as well as the feeding tubes and nasal oxygen cannulas. My girls still had a CPAP attached to their noses and a feeding tube down their throats, so the nurses had to make sure they positioned the babies on my chest in a way that they could still breathe and eat. They were on continuous feeds because their reflux was so bad.

This is not the way any new mother would like to carry their newborns for the first time. It was scary at first, but feeling my babies' skin on my skin for the first time was magical. I was traveling back to when they were both in my belly and all three of us were together. I lost sense of time and wasn't quite sure how long I had been in the NICU holding my girls that day. The alarms started going off and they both started desaturating. My time was up. I had to put them back in the incubators.

I had to pump for their nutrition every three hours and freeze what I was able to pump for my girls. After about a month, my milk supply started to decrease. We couldn't afford to keep Thiago in daycare anymore since Ronaldo's work had slowed down and we did not count on my income anymore. It was more feasible to just keep him home with me. I was only able to see the girls for two to three hours each day, so my body started to fail on me. The breast milk stopped coming down. Thiago was not able to go inside the NICU and Ronaldo had to work, so I couldn't go to the NICU to see my babies until he came home from work.

Women who had uncomplicated pregnancies had their newborns at home and could hold them all day long. In my case, I had a schedule to be able to hold my babies. The days went by so slowly. The NICU doctors kept telling me it was going to take time. They were just too premature and needed to grow. I grew impatient. I could not wait until they were home.

Days turned into weeks.

The babies were growing slowly, but surely. Sophia was doing amazing. After a few weeks she had gained a lot of weight, was on room air, and starting to bottle feed. Her desaturations were normal for her age. The NICU was not concerned about Sophia's development.

Alessia, on the other hand, was way behind her sister. She kept desaturating her oxygen levels, even on oxygen. The nurses tried multiple times a day to feed her in a bottle, but every time she tried to eat, she would reflux, and her oxygen levels desaturated. The nurses started getting concerned she was silently aspirating. The NICU doctors ordered a feeding therapist to come work with Alessia every day. At the time, I was still confident she was going to master the goal of eating. She just needed time. I would call the NICU multiple times a day to make sure the feeding therapist had stopped by. Every time I would go visit my babies, I would try to bottle feed Alessia and work with her swallow. No matter how hard we tried, she just could not coordinate her suck, swallow, and breathing reflexes.

On May 26, after forty-two days in the NICU, Sophia was ready to come home. It was a bittersweet feeling. I was happy that Thiago was finally going to meet one of his sisters and I was finally going to have one of my babies home. My mother had gotten Thiago a cute "Big Brother" T-shirt, which he was hesitant to wear at first. He was excited but shy. My mother waited with Thiago in the waiting room, while I went inside the NICU to go over discharge instructions. As soon as I saw my babies, I could not hold back my tears. The nurse must have gotten emotional too since she couldn't go through the discharge instructions without tearing up. She had taken care of Sophia for forty-two days.

I put my hands through the incubator opening and stroked Alessia's tiny body. I said to her, "I'm sorry you have to stay for a bit longer. You will come home soon—I promise. You just need to learn how to swallow and breathe. I love you." My heart was breaking. She was going to be alone without her sister. I felt so incredibly sorry for Alessia—I hated she was having so many struggles, and that I had to leave her at the hospital while I took Sophia home. But I didn't want Thiago to see me crying when I walked out of those NICU doors with Sophia. I went to the bathroom, washed my face, and came back to get Sophia. I hugged the NICU nurse and thanked her for everything. I placed Sophia in the car seat with all her bags on the hospital cart. I walked through the doors and my little Thiago was waiting. He was so excited. He couldn't believe his eyes when he saw his tiny little sister. He had waited so long to meet her. His eyes were glowing, he was so in love.

When we walked out of the hospital, Sophia's eyes started glimmering as she looked up at the blue sky. This was her first day breathing fresh air outside. As we drove away, my heart ached. All this will be over soon, I thought. Alessia will eventually join us at home, and I will never step foot in this hospital again. Little did I know that the Levine Children's Hospital would become my second home.

Sophia being at home brought me so much joy. Seeing her sweet face all the time and being able to hold her with no tubes or alarms sounding gave me a sense of normalcy as I put her in her crib, gave her baths, or took her out in her stroller. Unfortunately, Alessia was not progressing. She was not bottle feeding. She kept on throwing up and desaturating her oxygen levels. I began to lose hope that she would ever leave the NICU, and the doctors were starting to get concerned.

Two weeks after Sophia came home, a meeting was called in the NICU to discuss the plan for Alessia. The only things keeping her in the NICU were her inability to eat orally, her reflux, and oxygen desaturations. A placement of a feeding tube directly into her stomach, as well as a more complex airway evaluation and correction under general anesthesia was discussed. An ENT specialist had previously looked at her airway in the NICU and diagnosed her with a floppy airway called Laryngomalacia. Some premature babies have this floppy airway, caused by weak muscles. The walls of the airway collapse and compromise the airway, which in turn causes oxygen desaturations. Most kiddos improve with age or have surgery to correct the airway. The surgery for this consisted of shaving the excess tissue of the airway so that the walls wouldn't collapse and compromise the airway.

My sister, Jatrin, had come to my house to take care of Thiago and Sophia so I could spend more time with Alessia at the hospital and work with her swallow. I wanted Alessia to learn how to eat orally so badly, but I was starting to grow impatient. I wanted Alessia home. I agreed to the feeding tube placement surgery, hoping that she would come home, and I could work with her bottle feeding around the clock. She would master eating once she was home, I was sure of it. The surgery was scheduled for June 9.

I walked beside Alessia's hospital crib as they wheeled it towards the OR. I was shattered in a million pieces. She was only two months old and having her first surgery. I hated she was being put through this. It took time to accept the fact she was going to have a PEG tube in her stomach for nutrition. But the PEG tube was just the first step. After a few months, the PEG tube would get replaced with a G tube, or Mic-Key button (a more permanent feeding tube without the large extension the PEG tube had attached to it). In my mind, I was sure we would eventually not need the Mic-Key button.

When we arrived in the OR, I kissed her tiny little cheeks, said a prayer, and went to the waiting room with tears in my eyes.

Two hours went by. Two hours of uncontrollable anxiety. My mind raced. I was nervous, worried, and had a gut-wrenching feeling in my stomach. I lost count as to how many times I went to the bathroom. I paced from one side of the waiting room to the other. I prayed so hard.

Finally, they called my name. They put me in the conference room and told me the doctor would be in shortly. The procedure was complete. Thank God.

I was expecting the doctor to tell me, "She did extremely well. We inserted the PEG tube without complications, and we were able to correct her airway."

But no.

The doctor came in the conference room, sat down, and said, "We weren't able to insert the PEG tube, because to insert the breathing tube we had to pump air into her body, and the large intestine got in the way between the abdominal wall and the stomach. We are going to try to place the PEG tube tomorrow. She will have to remain sedated and intubated overnight." The doctor continued, "We also discovered that the floppiness of Alessia's airway goes all the way down to her lungs, so unfortunately it is not correctable with surgery. Hopefully with time it will correct itself, but we are concerned she might have a neurological issue going on in her brain that is causing this in her airway, and if that's the case, it may not get better, and she might need a tracheostomy in the future. We are scheduling an MRI either tonight or tomorrow to study her brain. We are hoping it will give us some clues to explain the anatomy of her airway, and the microtia ear."

My heart sank to the floor. The rest of what the doctor said was a blur. I couldn't make sense of what he was telling me. Anger, worry, frustration, and betrayal flooded through me. Anger that my prayers were not answered. Worry about the results of the MRI, which might show she did have a neurological problem. Frustration that they couldn't do anything surgically that day. Betrayal by God and at life. Life was preparing me for heartbreak that day.

I left the hospital, went home, and continued to pray.

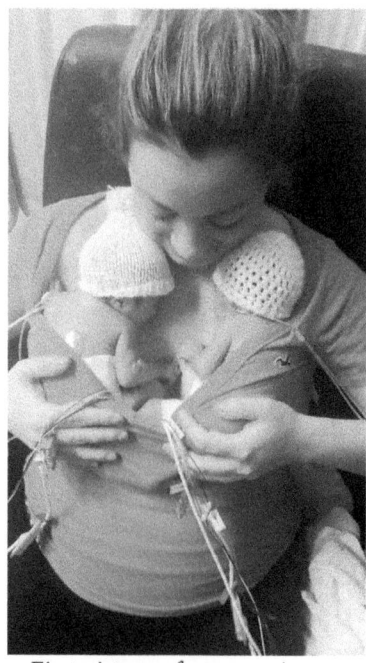
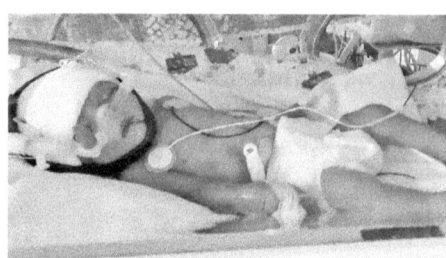

*Alessia Cruz, April 2015, Levine NICU*
*Photo Credit: Stephanie Detjen Costabel*

*First picture of me carrying my twins, April 2015. Levine NICU*
*Photo Credit: Lindsey Cook Howe*

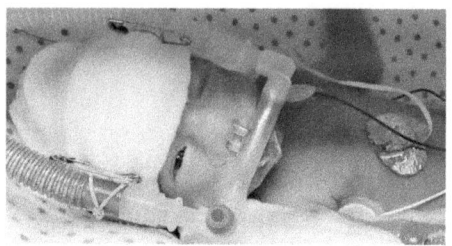

*Sophia Cruz, April 2015, Levine NICU*
*Photo Credit: Stephanie Detjen Costabel*

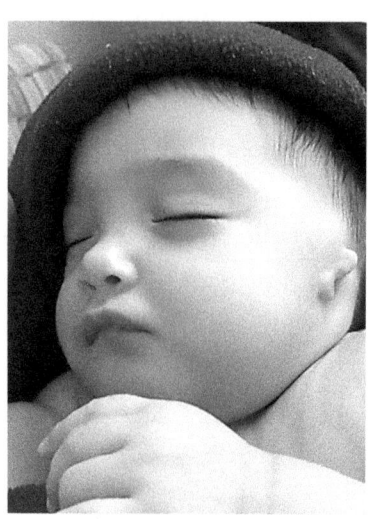
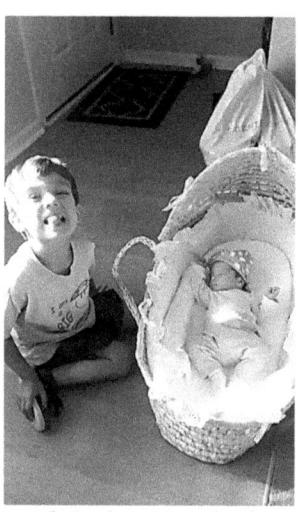

*Alessia's Microtia ear.*
*Photo Credit: Stephanie Detjen Costabel*

*Thiago with Sophia. First day home from the NICU, May 2015*
*Photo Credit: Stephanie Detjen Costabel*

# 5

I waited by the phone the following morning. Every time the phone rang my heart would skip a beat thinking it was the doctor. My hands were sweaty and cold. I called the NICU about fifty times throughout the morning, "Have you heard about Alessia?" I asked. "Is she still in surgery?" "Was the MRI completed?" Same questions every time I called.

"We haven't gotten any news from PACU, Mrs. Costabel; we promise to call you back as soon as we know she is out of surgery," the NICU nurse said. I felt my heart was going to come out of my chest. After a few hours, the phone rang and this time I knew it was the doctor. She had been in surgery since 8 a.m., and it was already 1 p.m. I was so relieved when I heard the doctor's voice. "Alessia has finished the procedure and is currently in recovery," he said. "The PEG tube was placed successfully on her stomach." *What a relief!* I thought. *Thank you, God.* My heart rate was returning to normal. "We also have the results of the MRI, and it shows some abnormalities."

My breathing started feeling uncomfortable. I could feel the anxiety overwhelming my body.

"She has an extremely rare malformation of her cerebellum called Rhombencephalosynapsis," he said.

*Oh my God. Is she going to be quadriplegic? Is she going to die? What the hell is this long word?* I thought. I noticed his stuttering when he said the word. He couldn't even pronounce the word right.

Sweat started dripping from my forehead. "What does this mean?" I asked him.

"Her cerebellum did not separate as it should have while being formed in the womb. Her cerebellum appears fused, and she does not appear to have a fully formed vermis."

I did not understand a word he was saying. "What exactly does this mean? Is this bad?" I asked.

"Well . . . this is a rare deformity. It may cause her to have developmental delays in a wide spectrum of areas—coordination of muscles, movement, processing information, speech, thinking, motor function, to name a few . . . I have called Neurology so they can come see her. I will have them call you to go more in detail as soon as they come to the NICU," he said.

More bad news, I thought. I thanked him for the call and hung up. I spelled this word on the Google search bar—Rhombencephalosynapsis—and clicked search. I could feel my heart in my throat. I was nauseated as I watched the ceiling begin to spiral in circles.

*Rhombencephalosynapsis: an abnormality of the cerebellum characterized by the absence of the vermis and continuity of the cerebellar hemispheres, dentate nuclei, and superior cerebellar peduncles. It either occurs as an isolated anomaly (rare) or as part of wider cerebral malformation and it has variable degrees of neurological impairment.*

I continued reading, skipping the words I did not understand.

*Clinical presentation includes truncal and/or limb ataxia, abnormal eye movements, head stereotypies, delayed motor development, and other features determined by supratentorial abnormalities. Overall patients tend to die in childhood or early adult life.*

I couldn't feel my fingers from the numbness. The words on the screen became blurry. It can't be true, I thought. I had to put the phone down before I threw up. My whole body was shaking.

I wanted to scream. I wanted to run as fast as I could to escape what I had just read. My heart ached, and I thought I was going to pass out. I panicked at the thought of my daughter dying. This could not be true.

I couldn't resist the urge to keep researching and opened Google again. I kept on scrolling, hoping to find an article that would have more positive information. I went into Facebook, hoping I would find more updated information. As I typed Rhombencephalosynapsis in the search bar, I trembled hoping I would find something, anything that would give me hope.

I came across a group called RES-trigeminal anesthesia. In parentheses it said Rhombencephalosynapsis. They had abbreviated that long word. RES, I thought, much easier to pronounce than Rhombencephalosynapsis. My heart rate came down. I filled out the questionnaire and asked to join. I clicked refresh every five minutes hoping I would be approved. Minutes went by like hours. All that I had read on Google gave such a grim prognosis. It wasn't fair.

Within an hour, I was approved to be a part of the group. I scrolled through and I saw pictures of smiling children, some in wheelchairs, and some standing. Many posts of proud mothers with the hashtag #TakethatRES showing off a mastered skill from their child skating, riding a bike, walking, running, using scissors to cut, writing, and even swimming. I saw photos of adults with RES. I sighed with relief. I could finally breathe. It may not be so bad after all, I thought.

I messaged the administrator, who was a mother of an RES kiddo. I asked her to please call me, since I was devastated with what I read on Google. I wanted to know what Rhombencephalosynapsis meant in terms of development and life prognosis. I prayed she would tell me my daughter wouldn't die.

She called me within an hour. "OMG!" she said. "You are the second person today that just found with their newborn twins, that one of them has RES! Please know that this isn't as scary from what you find in Google. I have an eight-year-old son with RES. We have quite a few very normal kiddos in the group. You will learn so much more from this group than any doctor or Google search." She sounded well-educated and knowledgeable about RES. "Please don't worry. Many children with RES do go on to adulthood." Thank God, I thought. I didn't let her finish her sentence before I nervously asked about RES and life prognosis.

"We have had some losses due to Chiari malformation and some intestinal issues," she said.

"Chiari? What the hell is that?" I asked. Clearly, I wasn't understanding the medical terminology.

"So, Chiari is when a part of the cerebellum dips into the spinal cord . . . by it going down into the spinal cord, there is pressure on the brain stem, which is what controls your respiratory reflexes. Did they mention anything to you about Chiari in her MRI?" she asked.

"No, not at all, I was told she only had Rhombencephalosynapsis," I replied.

"Well, Chiari is tricky . . . sometimes it's hard to see in a regular MRI. You might see a little portion of the cerebellum dipping through the spinal canal, but to actually see the severity of it, the best diagnosis test would be a flexion extension MRI," she said.

She continued, "There is also one more thing that is extremely important for you to know. There is a trigeminal anesthesia portion of the diagnosis. These kiddos don't perceive pain like normal people do. A lot of them have what is known as Gomez-Lopez-Hernandez Syndrome, which means they have trigeminal anesthesia. A lot cannot feel pain in the eyes and the face and have a very high pain tolerance in other areas of the body," she said.

"Well, that isn't really bad, right? That they don't feel pain?" I asked.

"Not necessarily. The human body needs to feel pain in order to heal certain wounds, to avoid danger, especially when it comes to the corneas."

I didn't want to continue bombarding her with questions, so I thanked her for the information and hung up. Now I had hope. The reassurance that Alessia might not die was enough for my body to feel normal again. My eyes were tired from crying, as well as my brain from thinking. I was exhausted, but relieved I had found this group and that I had spoken to another mother that had a child with RES. I took a shower to refresh my face and body, grabbed my purse, and drove to the hospital to see my sweet Alessia.

As I was driving to the hospital, I noticed how crystal blue the sky was. It was a sunny, hot, summer day in the middle of June. I put the windows down to feel the breeze while I drove. Looking at the sky and breathing the fresh air was calming. It will be okay, I thought. My sweet Alessia will grow into a beautiful woman. She will learn how to eat, talk, and walk. I know she will be just fine.

I walked through the hospital doors and stopped to marvel at the crystals hanging from the ceiling of the lobby. The sunlight reflected on these diamond shapes through the glass windows creating a rainbow of colors on the floor. It was a lovely sight. What an amazing hospital Levine Children's is, I thought. Alessia was so lucky to be in this hospital. Levine was the best pediatric hospital in the area, so I was thankful she was getting the best of care.

I took the elevator to the NICU recovery floor. After surgery, the babies are sent to recover at the NICU recovery, so she was not going to be in her usual spot. To go into the NICU, you must go through the cleaning station. They want to make sure no germs get in the NICU, so you had to wash your hands as well as put on a plastic gown so the germs on your clothes would not hurt the babies. I went through the cleaning station, anxious to see my sweet Alessia.

As soon as I walked in the NICU, I looked to my left and saw a baby. The baby was very swollen. I took a closer look at the baby, but this was not Alessia. Thank God, I thought. The poor baby was struggling so hard to breathe. It had a high flow CPAP, but its respiratory rate was high. The cheeks were so inflamed you could hardly see its eyes. It looked so uncomfortable and in pain. Poor baby, I thought. I felt sorry for its mother.

I kept walking through the NICU looking for Alessia. I went up to each baby, looking for Alessia's name. As I looked at them, I couldn't help thinking about how incredibly brave they were. So young and with so many struggles. Life is so unfair. There were about ten babies in the NICU, but I could not find my Alessia. That's odd, I thought, maybe I'm in the wrong area.

I approached one of the NICU nurses because I was beginning to worry. What if something had happened to her? "Excuse me," I said. "I am looking for my daughter Alessia Cruz—she just came out of a PEG tube surgery and MRI . . . not sure if I'm in the right area or not. She just came from recovery."

"Oh yes," she said, "she's right over there," and pointed to the swollen baby I saw when I walked in.

My heart started pounding. "No," I said, "that's not my baby! It does not look like my Alessia!"

"Yes, it is," she said. "She is very swollen from surgery and is having a hard time breathing after they extubated her."

My heart felt like it was going to rip out of my chest. I couldn't breathe. I started sobbing. I demanded to speak to the doctor. I walked over to the baby. This can't be her. It doesn't even look like her. I couldn't control my anxiety. The nervousness and despair I felt was leading me into a full-blown panic attack.

The nurse approached me and said, "Calm down, it's okay. This is expected after extubating, but she is fine, don't worry."

I was drowning in my tears. Finally, the doctor approached me and said, "Hi, Mrs. Costabel! Alessia's airway is very inflamed and irritated from the breathing tube. She is breathing this fast because her airway is very swollen and is being compromised. We are trying to avoid having to put her back on the breathing tube. I have ordered a course of steroids to help with the inflammation to bring the swelling down. The steroids will help with her breathing."

"She looks so uncomfortable," I said. "Is there anything we can do for this? Can I at least hold her and try to comfort her?"

"She is too unstable right now to be held, but we can certainly try swaddling her to see if it helps. She just got a dose of morphine, so we're just waiting for it to kick in; the steroids are also going to help her be more comfortable," she said.

My baby's fragile little body had a PEG tube inserted into her stomach. I wanted to pick her up and hug her and tell her how sorry I was, but I couldn't. She was trying so hard to breathe. She couldn't even cry because she couldn't breathe comfortably. Her arms and legs were wiggling, trying to self-soothe. I couldn't even see her eyes because her cheeks were so swollen. Why, God, do you allow such distress in a tiny little baby? I thought.

There was nothing I could do to help her. I just had to wait and hope the steroids would help her breathing and the pain medicine would help her pain. All I could do was pray and hope God would answer my prayers.

I stayed with her for a few hours, her condition not improving, until I had to get home to my other two children. It felt like I had a knife in my head from all the tension in my body.

That night, I could not remove the image of my poor baby in distress from my mind and could not stop sobbing. The NICU nurse must have known how devastated I was, and she called me later that evening with the news that the steroids and pain medications had worked: Alessia was more comfortable. I thanked her for letting me know and lay back against the pillow.

I hugged my pillow and said to myself, "It will get better. It has to."

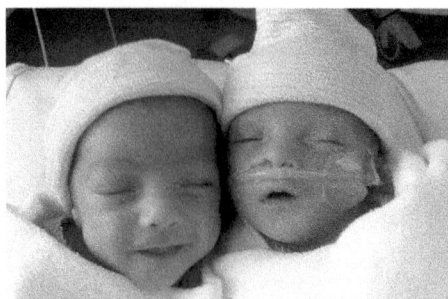

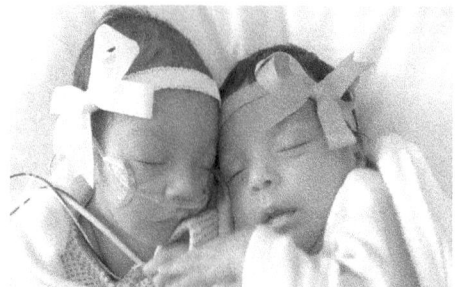

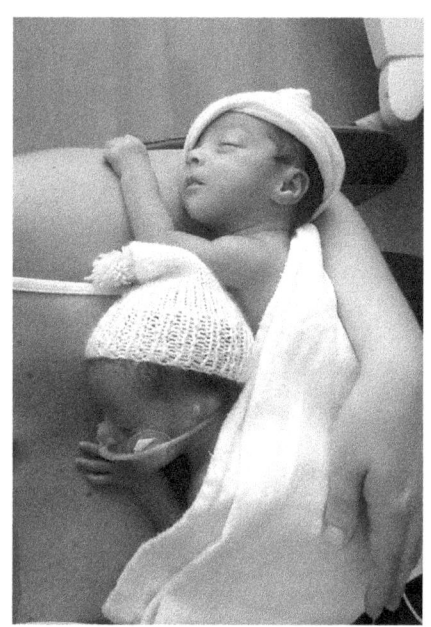

*The girls in the NICU, May 2015*
*Photo Credit: Stephanie Detjen Costabel*

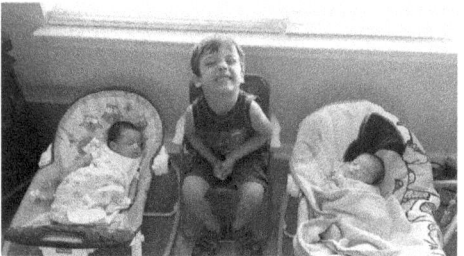

*Thiago with Sophia and Alessia the day Alessia came home. Photo Credit: Stephanie Detjen Costabel*

# 6

As the days went by, more tests were ordered for Alessia…

With the diagnosis of Rhombencephalosynapsis came many concerns from her medical team. Her swallow was uncoordinated, and her oxygen would dip every time she tried to swallow. They wanted to make sure she was able to swallow safely and was not silently aspirating.

Unfortunately, the swallowing test revealed she was silently aspirating her own secretions. Feeding therapy was placed on hold. We were not allowed to give her anything to eat by mouth. We were, however, allowed to use a pacifier to try and get her to suck on it so her swallowing muscles would learn to coordinate the suck, swallow, and breathe reflexes.

The failed swallowing test and the aspiration brought a whole new set of problems to the table. There was now a medical reason for her persistent reflux and oxygen desaturations. She choked on her own saliva every time she tried to swallow and then aspirated some of her reflux. She was put on reflux medication, but it wasn't helping. She was on continuous feeds and still threw up. The doctors were concerned she would end up developing aspiration pneumonia. Pulmonology and ENT were called in for their opinion. They discussed the possibility of needing to place a tracheostomy (an opening created in the front of the neck so a tube can be inserted into the windpipe to help you breathe) in the future if she started to develop too many aspiration pneumonias.

My lips quivered and my eyes filled with tears at the thought of Alessia needing a trach. I had to remain positive, I kept thinking to myself. Maybe she'll outgrow this. Maybe she'll eventually learn how to swallow safely. She just needed time. I couldn't bear the thought of another tube going into her body.

I offered her a pacifier every single second she was awake. I celebrated when Alessia was able to suck the pacifier more than once and not have an oxygen desaturation. After the third suck, though, she would desaturate and throw up. One day, she would suck the pacifier four times in a row, and other days she wasn't even able to hold it in her mouth. "She will move one step forward and ten steps back," the NICU team kept telling me. "Just keep offering her the pacifier."

A few days after the swallowing test came the hearing test. I walked into the NICU on an early Monday morning to speak to the audiologist that was going to conduct the hearing test. I walked over to Alessia's area and yawned. I had been up since 4 a.m. with Sophia. She had had a rough night not sleeping. Everyone was quiet. Wow, Mondays must affect the preemies just like adults, I thought.

Alessia's nurse greeted me, "Hi, Mrs. Costabel! They are just finishing up the hearing test. Alessia slept through the whole test. She had a rough night last night."

My eyes got big. "What happened?" I asked.

"Nothing too bad. Her reflux was just giving her a hard time. She seemed very fussy throughout the night. I'm actually glad she was able to finally fall asleep and get some rest," she said. "I'm glad you're here. The audiologist would like to go over the hearing test results with you."

I looked over to Alessia and saw the audiologist standing next to her crib, putting away all the hearing testing probes.

"Hi, Mrs. Costabel. I am Dr. Schneider, nice to meet you," she said.

"Nice to meet you too!" I quickly responded.

"We just finished her hearing test and found some unusual results."

*Oh God, what now?* I thought.

"We were thinking that on her right side of her face where she has a fully developed ear, she would have some sound responses. However, she did not respond to any of the thresholds that we tested her for. This implies that she is profoundly hearing-impaired in her right ear. Unfortunately, there isn't much to do on the right ear. Her hearing loss on this side is so severe that she would not benefit from hearing aids." She took her glasses off to clean them.

My heart started racing, thinking about a new hurdle for my baby.

"Good news is that on the left side, which is the side where she has her microtia (underdeveloped ear), she has a very mild hearing loss. Obviously since she doesn't have her ear canal, she does have a maximum conductive hearing loss. What this means is that what she hears is not clear, kind of like speaking under the water, since she has skin and bone between the outside world and her cochlea. She would need what is known as a bone anchored hearing aid, or BAHA for short. It is a hearing aid that goes on a headband. Sound travels through her bone to her cochlea. I will refer you to the audiologist who does those hearing aid fittings. It may take a couple of months to get approved through Medicaid, but once she gets that hearing aid, her hearing on that side should be very close to normal," she said. Thank God for Medicaid, I thought. Thankfully, with all Alessia's disabilities we qualified for Medicaid for the Disabled.

"Well, that's ironic," I said. "You would think she would hear on the side she actually has an ear . . . shows how physical appearance is nothing. You can have a perfectly formed ear, but if it's hearing impaired it is useless."

"Yes indeed," Dr. Schneider replied.

The fact that she would need a hearing aid didn't bother me at all. I was relieved that she had at least some hearing. I just didn't understand how it was possible you could hear without an ear on one side, and on the other side where you do have an ear you are profoundly deaf.

As I watched my baby sleeping, I wondered how incredibly rare she was. She was comfortable, sound asleep all curled up in a little ball. Her mouth was partially opened, her eyes halfway shut. She smiled in her sleep and then frowned. Her lips twitched as if trying to suck. I couldn't help noticing how cute her tiny microtia ear looked.

I felt a tap on my shoulder. "Hi, Mrs. Costabel." It was the feeding therapist that had come to work with Alessia's oral skills. "Oh, wow, she finally fell asleep!" she said as she looked over to Alessia's crib. "I had come earlier to work with her, but she was inconsolable. I'm going to let her rest for now. I do want to talk to you about something that I've noticed when we work on her sucking on her pacifier."

Oh Lord, I thought. Please don't let it be bad.

"I have noticed that her left jaw is very tight," she said. "She can't really open that side of her mouth that much. I brought a special oral stimulation brush called a NUK brush so we can work on opening that side of her mouth more. It's just very tight. The NUK brush has a rubber side with texture on it that will help open her mouth up more. I think the more we help open it up, she'll loosen up a little. Nothing to worry about right now, though! I'll come back later when she's awake."

I sighed a breath of relief. Thankfully, it wasn't terrible news. I didn't have the energy to keep worrying. I didn't want anything distracting the immense love and joy I felt watching my baby sleep.

I took a picture of her sweet sleeping face, kissed her tiny pink cheeks, and went home. Sophia was already asleep. I lay next to her and observed her sleeping face. She looked just as sweet and beautiful as her sister. I could feel the guilt creeping in on me. "I am so sorry I was gone all day, baby," I whispered in her ear. Ronaldo and Thiago were asleep too. I had lost track of time. I had been in the NICU the entire day. I cried myself to sleep that night. One day we will all be together, and this nightmare will end, I thought.

The following day, the doctor called me to give me some exciting news.

"Good morning, Mrs. Costabel!"

I could hear the enthusiasm in his voice.

"Alessia is close to going home, the PEG tube is in, and the tests have been completed. We just have to schedule a day where you can come and room in," he said.

I felt like a little girl on her birthday. I smiled from ear-to-ear. Finally! "That's amazing! Thank you so much! What exactly is 'room in'?" I asked.

"We have to make sure you feel comfortable with the feeding tube machine and with the overall care of Alessia with her PEG tube and her medical needs. We need to schedule a day where you can come and stay the night with her. We have rooms here and you would have your own room. You would use this night as a sample night to practice feeding and attending to her yourself."

"Can we do it this Friday?" I asked. It had to be a day when Ronaldo could stay with Sophia and Thiago so I could go and spend the night at the NICU. Fridays were usually slow for Ronaldo.

"Of course!" he responded. I couldn't wait. I was finally going to spend the night with my Alessia. Friday came around; check-in time was at 8 p.m. I pumped before I left to make sure Ronaldo had enough food for Sophia. I kissed my Thiago and Sophia and headed for the hospital. This will be some much-needed mommy-daughter time, I thought. I knew Alessia would be so comfortable sleeping with me. She needed to be next to her mother.

I checked into the NICU and was led to my room. A queen-size bed, I thought. Wow, we are going to sleep so well here tonight! It was cozy.

The dim lights made it feel like a hotel room.

The nurse came in. "Okay, I'm about to bring Alessia over. I have the alarm there where you can ding me if you need me. There's also a camera over there just in case," she said as she pointed to the far-right corner of the ceiling. "We do ask that you do not sleep with the baby because of the risk of SIDS."

Are you fucking kidding me? I thought. I have been waiting for nine weeks to sleep with my baby, to cuddle her, and you're telling me I can't sleep with my own baby? I could feel the fume coming out of my ears. I wasn't going to argue, though. It was too early in the night. I bit my tongue and just nodded.

The nurse brought Alessia in her crib with the feeding pump, the breast milk supply, and a special bag called a Farrell bag to capture the air that could come out of the feeding pump. I had pumped so much during the first month that I had a lot of frozen breast milk stored. The feeding pump was attached to an IV pole. The feeding bag ran through the feeding pump and was connected to her PEG tube in her stomach. Halfway down the line, there was another tube that was connected to the Farrell bag.

"Okay, we are all set," the nurse said. "The first thing you have to do is turn on the pump. Once the pump is turned on, you are going to prime the breast milk all the way down to the tip of the tube, right before reaching the bottom. You must make sure you prime the pump first, because if you don't, what you are going to be feeding Alessia is air. By priming it, you make sure the milk is all the way at the bottom, ready to go directly into her stomach. Breast milk is good for approximately two to three hours, so you want to make sure you put enough breast milk in the feeding bag to last you for two hours. After two hours, you must throw away whatever is left in the bag and add another two hours' worth of breast milk. Formula is good for four hours, so when you run out of breast milk and you start using the formula, then you will be able to change the milk every four hours. This is the button you press to prime the pump." She showed me how to prime the pump. "Once the milk has reached the end, then you connect it to the PEG tube that goes directly into her stomach."

Okay, that doesn't seem that hard, I thought. She had me practice a few times how to prime the pump. Once I mastered that technique of priming the pump we went on to the settings of the pump. "Okay . . . so because she has severe reflux, we have her on continuous feeds. Currently, she is on 15 MLS per hour for twenty-three hours of the day. Once she is able to tolerate this amount well without throwing up, then you can discuss with her GI doctor to see if her hourly feeds can be increased so she can be off the pump for a few hours," she said.

"So, she will have to be connected to this machine continuously for twenty-three hours a day?" I asked.

"Yes, for now she will." She continued with her instructions. "Now this over here sitting right next to the feeding bag is the Farrell bag." She pointed to an empty bag hanging next to the feeding bag. "This permits the gases from her stomach to escape. We don't want her to have too much air in her stomach because that will make her reflux worse and make her feel uncomfortable. The Farrell bag must be above her heart in order for it to work properly, so we usually hang it next to the feeding bag on the IV pole." She hung it on the pole. "If the Farrell bag is below her heart, then you risk all of her milk going to the Farrell bag instead of the stomach."

I frowned. This was going to be a process. She was going to have to be connected to this freaking pole. I would have to get used to carrying her and the pole. "Excuse me," I interrupted. "I am curious to know when exactly she will be able to go off of continuous feeds and not be connected to this machine. Do we have an estimate?" I asked.

She cleared her throat. "I am so sorry. I know this is all very difficult to process right now. I cannot answer that question for you. We hope her reflux will be under control in a few weeks and then you can start adding more MLSs to her hourly rate and get a couple of hours off the pump. But you will have to discuss that with Dr. Pineiro, her GI doctor," she replied. "It will all get easier once you get used to the feeding pump."

After she finished teaching me, she said, "All right, Stephanie, I hope you have a good night. Enjoy your baby. Please remember that in two hours you have to add more milk to the bag. Don't hesitate to give me a ring if you need me. The bell is right there next to your bed." I wanted to cling on to her legs. Please don't leave me! I thought. Now I was scared to be on my own with Alessia. This was a complicated process. Alessia slept throughout my whole training. I wanted to pick her up so badly, but she looked so comfortable sleeping that I decided to just wait until she woke up. Alessia's hospital crib had one IV pole connected to it that was the monitor connected to her heart rate, respiratory rate, and pulse oximeter leads. On the other pole was the feeding pump, feeding bag, and Farrell bag. All the tubes were secured together and went underneath her pajamas to prevent tangling. Now I was afraid to pick up my own daughter. God, I hope I do this well, I prayed.

After about an hour, she started moving. I started to panic. I didn't want to call the nurse because I had to prove that I was capable of taking care of my daughter without a nurse's help. I grabbed all the tubes with one hand and with the other hand I carefully picked Alessia up from her crib. I couldn't go very far because she was connected to all these tubes, and I didn't want any tube to be disconnected. I settled on the chair next to the crib. She started to cry. My hands started shaking. "What's wrong, Alessia?" I whispered. It wasn't time to change her milk. I still had two hours. I checked her diaper, it was dry. She kept crying. The monitor started to alarm. Her oxygen levels started to desaturate.

She started throwing up. I quickly sat her up a little so she wouldn't choke on her vomit. My hands trembled as I carefully changed her diaper and pajamas and cleaned the vomit off of her leads. At that point, she was screaming. "It's okay, baby," I whispered as I tried to comfort her. The crying eased up for a little bit as she tried to get comfortable in my arms. She was wiggly and let out a cry every couple of minutes. She was frowning, nervous. I got the impression she was not comfortable. I sat holding her in that chair for approximately two hours, and then the feeding pump started to beep. It was time to add more milk to the bag. She still hadn't gone back to sleep yet.

As I laid her down in her crib, I added more milk to the feeding bag and re-started the feeding pump. She started moaning and then cried. She would stop crying and a couple of minutes later start crying again. I looked at the clock as I yawned. Something was wrong. I could sense it.

I finally got the nerve to page the nurse. She quickly came in. "I'm so sorry," I said. "I just feel that something isn't right with Alessia. She hasn't slept. I've already changed her clothing after she had an event of reflux earlier. I've changed her feeding bag and put in more fresh milk. She is uncomfortable for some reason. Could you page the doctor, please?" I asked.

"Yes, of course," she replied. After about forty-five minutes, I heard a knock on the door. It was the doctor. Thank God, I thought. Alessia had yet to fall asleep. She had been very fussy. It was 4 a.m. and she had not slept for the past four hours. The doctor introduced himself. "Hi, Mrs. Costabel, I heard you have been having a rough night with Alessia," he said.

"Yes," I replied. "She is very uncomfortable. She has been crying and moaning on and off ever since she threw up about four hours ago."

"She may just be having a bad night," he said. "We already gave her reflux medication before you got here. The nurses have mentioned to me that she has been having restless nights. I wonder if we should get her on nerve pain medicine. A lot of kiddos that have neurological issues have nerve pain. We can try and see. Let me put an order in to start her on gabapentin, and let's observe her for the next couple of days and see if she is able to sleep better. Are you okay working the feeding pump?" he asked.

"Yes," I said. "It's not the feeding pump that worries me. It is the fact that she doesn't sleep and that she seems uncomfortable."

"Completely understandable," he said. "Let's put this order in and see how it goes." He excused himself and left the room. There was a moment in the night where I could not control my urge to sleep. I ended up falling asleep with Alessia in my arms. Her cries and moans would stop, and I would fall asleep. But then she would start crying and moaning again and I would wake up. That continued until the nurses switched shifts at 7 a.m.

It was time to go and Alessia was still awake. I couldn't keep my eyes open. I yawned more than I could blink. I wanted to be home and go to sleep. I was dizzy and light-headed from the lack of sleep. Alessia had spent the whole night awake. This couldn't be normal. The nurse came into the room to get Alessia and bring her back to the NICU.

"I'm very concerned," I said to the nurse. "I can't believe she is still awake. She has not slept since 11 p.m. last night and it's almost 8 in the morning."

"Yes, I think we are all concerned," the nurse replied. "I am about to give her the first dose of gabapentin, and hopefully that will get her to sleep. Go home and get some rest—I know it was a rough night for you. I'll call you in the afternoon with an update."

I'm not sure how I made it home. I was so tired. As soon as I walked into the house, I went straight to my room and passed out. I didn't even say hi to Thiago or Sophia. I didn't even ask Ronaldo how the night had gone. He asked me how it went, but I was so tired I didn't even reply. I could not keep my eyes open. I threw myself on my bed and fell into a deep sleep.

# 7

I was running through hallways. The darkness made me tremble. It was so cold I couldn't feel my fingers. In the distance I could hear her scream. I must be in the NICU. I frantically searched for anyone with scrubs. Where are the nurses? There was no one there. The solitude was frightening. The alarms went off, alerting that she had stopped breathing. I could hear her, but I could not see her. She was crying as she gasped for air. I ran from one room to the next. All of them were empty. Not a crib, not a baby, not a nurse, just empty rooms and hallways. My heart was about to come out of my chest. I felt dizzy. I held my balance by leaning on the walls. Suddenly there was silence. Alessia was no longer screaming, crying, or gasping for air. The monitors kept alarming. "SOMEBODY PLEASE HELP!" I screamed, frantic. "Where are you, Alessia?" My knees turned into jelly. I couldn't feel my body. My vision went pitch black as I fell to the ground.

I felt somebody shaking me. "Wake up! Wake up, baby!" I slowly opened my eyes as I watched the ceiling go in circles. It was Ronaldo. "Are you okay?" he asked as he caressed my cheek. "You've been screaming Alessia's name and kicking in your sleep . . . it was just a nightmare, baby," he said, as he wrapped his arms around me. I let out a sigh of relief. "Thank God that was just a dream," I murmured. "I could not find her. The rooms were empty. Baby, I couldn't find her!" I started to sob.

The following day I went to the NICU to see my Alessia. I found her fast asleep in her Mama Roo swing. She had a NICU nurse attending her who I hadn't met before. "Good morning, I'm mom." I dropped my backpack on the nearby chair. "Could you please page the doctor?" I asked.

"Yes, of course." She seemed empathetic, as if the whole NICU had already told her what a unique case Alessia's case was. I told her about my dream as I settled into the rocking chair next to Alessia.

"You know, it's common," she said, as she stopped the feeding pump to change Alessia's feeding bag. "A lot of mothers of preemies go through a lot of traumas with their babies here in the NICU. I can't even imagine your situation who has had two babies in the NICU, and one with complex needs. Hang in there." She patted my shoulder, trying to comfort me. The NICU nurses always understood. They had seen firsthand what I had been through. They had seen me cry, panic, smile, and laugh. They had seen me go through all kinds of emotions in the past two months.

"Good morning, Mrs. Costabel." I glanced over my shoulder; it was the NICU doctor.

"Oh, that was quick! I'm so glad you're here." I shook his hand. I hadn't met him before. He knew Alessia's case well and I had talked to him over the phone, but we had not ever crossed paths in the NICU. "I would like to know when my daughter could come home," I asked, a hopeful tone in my voice.

"I think she might be ready. We started her on gabapentin, and we just need to increase her dose to the dose that neurology has suggested. If she tolerates it well for the next 48 hours, then she should be good to go." I smiled from ear to ear. It was the best news I had received in weeks. I started tearing up. "We have ordered a pulse oximeter machine so you can take it home with you. You can monitor her oxygen levels at night while she sleeps, or whenever you feel she isn't breathing right," he said.

I wanted to hug him for this joyful news. It was happening. She was coming home.

The date was set, June 24: seventy-one days since her birth. Seventy-one days of agony every time they would call me to give me bad news. Seventy-one days of traveling back and forth from the NICU to my home. Seventy-one days stuck in a crib in the hospital without her family. Alessia was a brave fighter. I admired her strength.

It was a beautiful day for discharge—the perfect day for Alessia to come home. I had waited so long for that day I should have been clapping my hands and jumping up and down from the excitement, but honestly, I was terrified. The pulse oximeter machine, the feeding tube, and her complex medical needs frightened me. I didn't let it show, though.

My mother stayed with Thiago and Sophia at home, while Ronaldo and I drove to Levine to pick Alessia up. This would be the last time I would drive to Levine without my daughter, I thought. Or at least I hoped. The discharge took hours. I had to show them I was able to work the pulse oximeter machine, the feeding pump, and how to administer her medicines. The hole on her stomach where the PEG tube had been inserted had healed rather quickly, so I only needed to change the gauze around it twice a day. My palms were sweaty, and my hands shook while I administered her medicines through her feeding tube. But I hid my nervousness well. I did not want anything to stop the possibility of her coming home that day.

"Wow, it looks like you are a pro!" the nurse exclaimed. "You will be just fine. Alessia is in good hands."

After I proved myself competent of being Alessia's nurse and mother, the NICU finally discharged her. We put her in her car seat and hurried out of the NICU as if the NICU would stop her discharge. I was still in disbelief she was finally going home. Both Ronaldo and I walked out of those hospital doors with smiles on our faces. I had imagined Alessia would be happy to be outside too. But I couldn't tell if she really felt a difference of being outside in the warm weather.

As Ronaldo drove home, I sat in the back with her. This was the first day her face actually got some sun—she was very pale. I quickly looked at the oxygen monitor, terrified of her desaturating. Her oxygen levels were normal, in the 95-100 range. She had not had any reflux all morning. The feeding pump was working normally. I had attached the feeding pump and her Farrell bag to the hook in our van so it would be above her body. But she wasn't looking around—her expression was the same as when she was in the NICU. Maybe she doesn't really care too much to be outside, I thought. Maybe she is just tired.

When we pulled into the driveway, I saw Thiago waiting on the front porch. "They're here!" he shouted. He could not wait to meet Alessia. "Is this Alessia?" he asked. I nodded as I put the car seat down so he could see her.

"Hi, Miss Alessia," he said to her as he pulled her hat up a little to be able to kiss her cheek. "What's wrong with her ear?" he asked.

I was amazed at how Thiago always noticed the smallest details of things. It was the first thing he noticed.

"Does she have a broken ear, Mama? Is that why she was in the hospital for so long?" He was worried, and I could tell he felt sorry for his sister.

I giggled. "It's not broken, silly," I said as I stroked his cheek. "She's just like Nemo. Do you remember Nemo?" I asked. "Nemo had a very tiny fin. Alessia just has a very tiny ear. But it's okay. It's not broken. It works perfectly well," I assured him. "In fact, it's the only ear in which she can hear."

When we walked in, I laid Alessia's car seat right next to Sophia, who was lying comfortably in her baby rocker seat. I wanted to document this homecoming with a picture. "Thiago, will you sit on the couch? I'm going to put both of your sisters next to you so we can take a nice picture," I said. His eyes sparkled as he sat on the sofa with a smile from ear-to-ear.

I carefully picked Alessia up, fearing I might break her. Her body was so tiny—she was only five pounds. I laid her in one of Thiago's arms. I picked up Sophia next. What a difference four weeks with her had made!!!! I wasn't scared to break her. She was plumper than Alessia, and I was used to carrying her. I laid her next to Thiago in his other arm. I took the first picture of my three children together. My three children side-by-side. I was in love. I wanted to be in that moment forever—happy tears welled in my eyes. I will cherish that first picture for the rest of my days on this Earth.

We had quite the celebration. My mother, Ronaldo, and I were so relieved to have her at home that we all had a glass of white wine. No more trips to the hospital, I thought. I noticed Alessia and Sophia sleeping peacefully side by side on the sofa. I quickly took another picture with my phone. I wanted to capture every single joyful moment I witnessed of my sweet twin girls.

We had been so excited and nervous throughout the day that by nightfall, Ronaldo and I were exhausted. I had all my alarms ready for the night: every three hours, I would need to change the milk for the feeding bag. The breast milk that I had saved from my first month of pumping was all in the fridge, ready to be dumped into the feeding bag. All of Sophia's bottles with my breast milk were also prepared for the night. I was pumping the little breast milk I had left and mixing it with additional formula for two babies. I had two bassinets right next to our bed. It would be easier for me to attend to them if we were all close together. My mother and Ronaldo helped me get everything situated. What could possibly go wrong? It wasn't like I was alone, but the thought of not having the nurse nearby freaked me out a little. "Everything will be okay, everything is ready. Go to sleep while the girls are sleeping so you can rest some," my mom said as she kissed me good night and headed home. I wanted her to stay so badly, but knew she had to go home and get some rest; she had to work the next day.

By 9 p.m., I was in bed and trying to get some sleep. It would be time to feed Sophia in two hours and change Alessia's feeding bag in three hours. The pulse oximeter machine was reading normal for Alessia's oxygen levels. The feeding pump was doing its job feeding her. The girls looked comfortable and were sound asleep. I drifted off for a solid two hours.

I was woken up by Sophia's cries for food. She needed feeding like clockwork. Every two to three hours, she was up to eat. She had an amazing appetite. Ronaldo went to warm up her bottle, while I changed her diaper.

Suddenly Alessia's pulse oximeter machine started alarming of a desaturation. I looked at the numbers reflecting on the screen . . . 88 . . . 87 . . . 86 . . . 70 . . . My heart started racing. My hands began shaking as I started tapping Alessia's back to wake her up a little to breathe. She opened her eyes, started gasping for air, burped, and threw up. Her oxygen levels started to increase: 86 . . . 88 . . . 90 . . . 95 . . . she was back at baseline. Phew! I breathed a sigh of relief. It was evident her reflux was causing her desaturations. I stopped the feeding pump, disconnected everything, cleaned her vomit, and changed her. She had thrown up quite a bit . . . probably most of her feed from the past two hours.

She was crying, frantic. I held her for about an hour without any tubes connected to her. I felt comfortable holding my baby normally without worrying about all the tubes for that one hour. I felt she could be off the feeding tube for an hour to give her tummy a break. I had seen the nurses do it after she had a bad reflux episode. I can't wait until all these tubes are out of the picture, I thought, frustrated and in tears.

Ronaldo had already fed Sophia and put her back to sleep. It would be another two hours before she would wake up again for another bottle, but Alessia still had not gone back to sleep. She whimpered and cried as if something was bothering her. I handed her over to Ronaldo while I got her reflux medication. I had already given her gabapentin and that should have relieved any nerve pain she might have had. It had to be the reflux. I gave her the medicine through her PEG tube, got her feeding pump ready, switched out her milk from the feeding bag, laid her next to me, and prayed she would fall asleep. I glanced at the clock as I yawned. It was already 2 a.m. Sophia would wake up in an hour and at 5 a.m. I would have to switch out Alessia's feeding bag again. Ugh. Then at 6 a.m. Sophia would wake up again to eat. If she even made it to six. I couldn't keep my eyes open. The need to sleep started making me grumpy. I started crying softly, thinking how incredibly hard this was. Premature twin babies and one on a feeding tube. My poor Thiago would have to see me in a terrible mood from my lack of sleep.

I glanced over to my husband hoping he would comfort me, but the poor thing was passed out. He had to work the following day and had to get some rest. The worried thoughts kept racing through my head, and although I was incredibly tired, I was also emotionally restless. I glanced at the clock for the fiftieth time—2:45 a.m.—Sophia was already starting to move. Might as well go ahead and feed her, I thought. Hopefully, I can sleep from 3 a.m. to 5 a.m. I got up and got Sophia's bottle and sat it on my nightstand. She let out one cry and I immediately gave her the bottle. I looked over to Ronaldo and he hadn't moved. He was so fast asleep he didn't hear her. I rolled my eyes, envious of his deep sleep, and irritated. By 3:30 a.m. Sophia was fed, burped, changed, and back to sleep. Alessia was sound asleep too. I had one and a half hours before I had to change Alessia's feeding bag. This is my chance, I thought. I drifted off to sleep.

In the distance, I could hear a beeping noise. It was so annoying. It wouldn't stop. I don't know how long the beating lasted, but I thought I was dreaming. I woke up startled and realized it was the feeding pump beeping. It was time to change the feeding bag. I glanced at the clock. It was 5:30 a.m. Still halfway asleep, I got up and changed the feeding bag. Alessia was still asleep, and her oxygen levels were normal. Thank God she hadn't thrown up. I probably should change her diaper, I thought while I tried to keep my eyes opened. I lay back on my bed and drifted back to sleep again.

This time I was awakened by Sophia's cries for food. It was 6:30 a.m. My hungry baby. I was hardly able to move from exhaustion. Ronaldo had slept through it all. I shook him gently. "Baby, please feed Sophia—I need to sleep. I have two hours before I have to change Alessia's feeding bag." He slowly got up to realize it was already morning.

It seemed like I was asleep for just half an hour before I started hearing Thiago's little voice. "Good morning, Mama, what are we going to do today?" he asked, so cute and excited.

Ugh . . . the exhaustion felt unbearable, and it was only the first night. How am I ever going to get some sleep? Thank God there's coffee and Ronaldo hadn't left for work yet. I yawned and put the covers above my head. It was 8 a.m. and I was clearly not ready to start my day.

# An Amazing Little Girl with Rhombencephalosynapsis

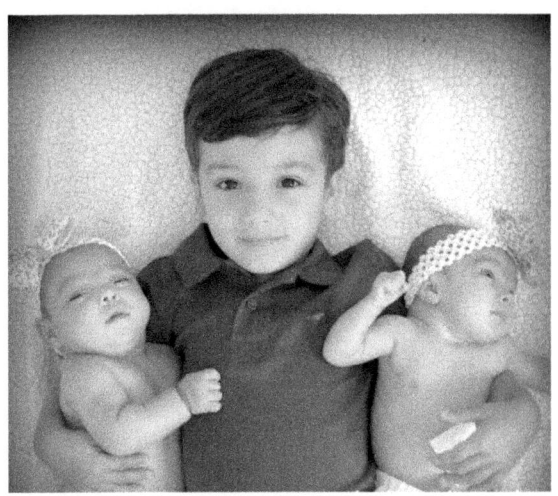

*Thiago with Sophia and Alessia, June 2015*
*Photo Credit: Jody Williams Photography*

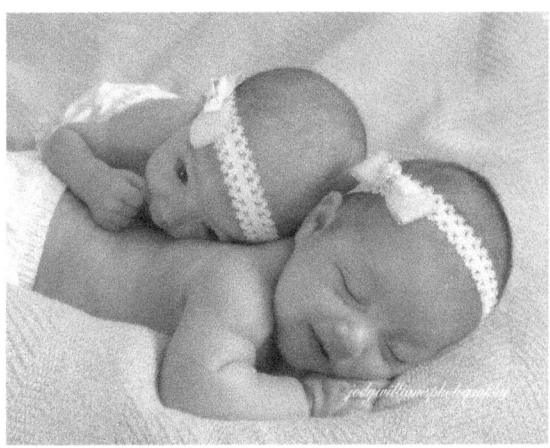

*Sophia and Alessia, June 2015*
*Photo Credit: Jody Williams Photography*

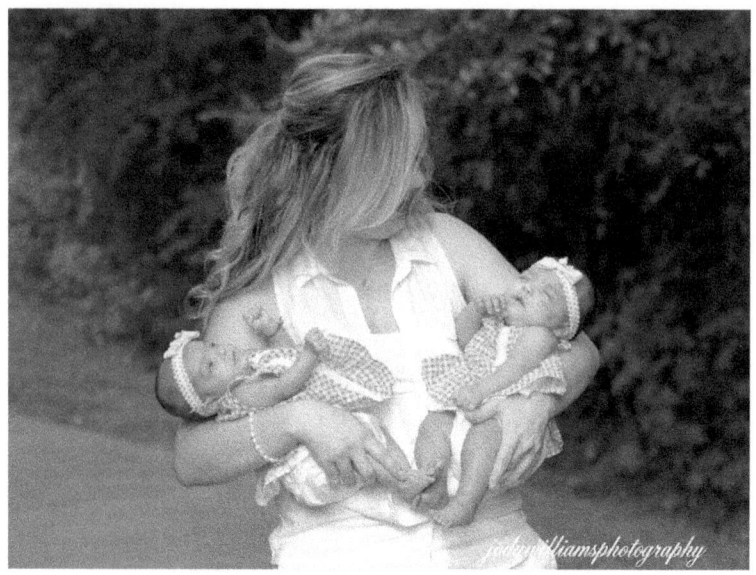

*Sophia, Alessia, and me, June 2015*
*Photo Credit: Jody Williams Photography*

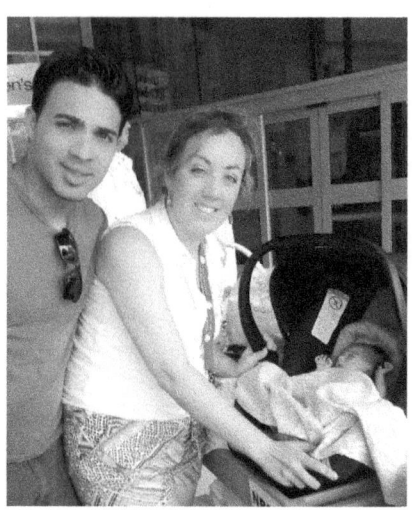

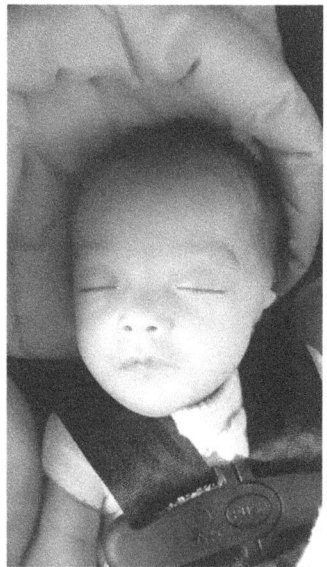

*Alessia heading home!!!*
*Photo Credit: Cristina Costabel*

# 8

The days went by, and I felt like I was on a 24-hour nurse shift with little breaks in between. I had come to completely master Alessia's medical machines. I didn't tremble anymore every time a machine beeped or alarmed. But it was hard for any of us to get much sleep with the pulse oximeter machine alarming throughout the night. Alessia's reflux was still desaturating her oxygen levels, but once she vomited, her oxygen levels would go back to normal, so I wasn't as worried as I had once been.

When you have a baby with disabilities you immediately qualify for Early Intervention—a service group that offers Physical, Occupational, and Speech Therapy for NICU graduates with developmental delays. Early intervention would call me every day. I dreaded those calls. Not that they weren't being helpful, but they seemed to always call when I had a chance to grab a nap, usually mid-morning when both girls were asleep, and Thiago was in preschool. Alessia needed physical, occupational, feeding, and hearing therapy. They all needed to come once a week for one-hour sessions for each therapy. It seemed like I had a therapist in my house every day. They were all there to help Alessia and me with Alessia's developmental goals, but I was beyond exhausted those first couple of weeks—the only help I desired was a chance to sleep. We also had a nurse that would come once a week to check all Alessia's vital signs and make sure she was gaining weight. She had a friendly personality and gave me a sense of security.

Then came all the follow-up appointments. She had seven different specialists to follow up with after her discharge from the NICU. Audiology, Genetics, Pulmonology, GI, ENT, Neurology, and Pediatrician.

I was given an extensive list of pediatric clinics to choose from, but I was so exhausted from my lack of sleep that I didn't care to research any of them. Thiago's pediatrician was forty minutes away from my house at the time. It wasn't bad since he was healthy and didn't often require follow-ups. But with the girls, I had to pick someone closer. I turned to the last page and picked the last one on the list, Walker Pediatrics. The name sounded simple, so I chose it without thinking much of it. I longed for simplicity and normalcy.

This was the first time I was taking Alessia out after being home from the NICU. The preparation of getting both girls ready for the doctor's appointment was an ordeal. Between Sophia's bottles, changes of clothing, Alessia's pulse oximeter machine, feeding pump, feeding bags, syringes, diapers, wipes, and double stroller, I hardly had much time left to get ready myself. Thank God Ronaldo had taken the day off to stay with Thiago and help me get the girls ready. But even with his help it took a lot longer than I had anticipated.

Yes, I was still in pajamas. I quickly went up to the bathroom to change and looked in the mirror. I looked terrible—I hadn't noticed until now. Between attending to Sophia and managing Alessia's medical needs, I had completely forgotten about myself. The dark circles under my eyes looked like I hadn't slept in years. My wardrobe now consisted of day and night pajamas.

The girls' pediatrician appointment was at 10 a.m., and it was already 9:40, and I still needed to drive downtown. I hurried to try and find something to wear, breaking into a sweat. No time to shower, I cleaned myself with baby wipes. I quickly washed my face and threw on the first thing I found in my closet. I ran out the door with the two girls securely fastened in their car seats.

I monitored the girls through the rearview mirror. Sophia's eyes were halfway shut as she yawned. She always enjoyed a nice car ride and would be asleep in no time. I was thankful she was so easy— Sweet Sophia never gave any trouble as long as she was fed. It was like she knew that my hands were so busy with Alessia's medical needs. I glanced over to Alessia and noticed her color looked off. Her cheeks were not pink anymore. She was of a grayish color, like the oxygen in her blood was low. I didn't have the pulse oximeter machine connected to her leads, so I was unable to see her actual oxygen levels. I was ten minutes from the clinic.

My heart raced, then I heard her burp and throw up on her brand-new outfit that Jatrin had gotten her the week before. I kept glancing at her through the rearview mirror while I looked for a place to stop, but I was in the middle of the highway. Luckily, as soon as she threw up, her face slowly began turning pink again. She is aspirating every time she refluxes, I thought. I remembered what her pulmonologist had said in the NICU about the possibility of needing a tracheostomy: "As long as she does not develop aspiration pneumonia."

I turned on the street where the clinic was located. It was already 10:20 a.m. I was twenty minutes late and I still had to change Alessia out of her dirty clothes.

Once safely inside, we met Dr. Jennifer Squires—a charming, young woman. She had recently started her medical career and had the burst of energy of a brand-new pediatrician. She was exactly the pediatrician Alessia needed. She did not have much experience with children with Rhombencephalosynapsis, but she was eager and motivated to find any information that could be of use to us. I had previously called the clinic to discuss Alessia's diagnosis to make sure her doctor knew about her.

Dr. Squires was on top of everything. She had contacted the University of Washington's research team dedicated to Rhombencephalosynapsis and Gomez Lopez Hernandez syndrome prior to our appointment. Her eyes glowed when she handed me over an email from Dr. Doherty, the head of the RES research at UW. Dr. Squires helped us enroll in the research program. Being that RES was a rare diagnosis, they were interested in every child diagnosed with this brain malformation, along with their families. I was extremely impressed at Dr. Squires's motivation and desire to help us understand more about the disease and what it would entail in Alessia's future.

"Her head circumference is within normal limits," Dr. Squires said cheerfully, "we just have to keep an eye on it because of her high risk of developing hydrocephalus." I remembered that the RES mom from Facebook had mentioned to me that a lot of children with RES are born with hydrocephalus—a build-up of fluid in the brain—or end up developing it later in life. Alessia's ventricles were slightly larger than normal, but not concerning yet, and I desperately hoped it would remain that way. "When is your follow-up appointment with GI?" she asked. She was concerned about Alessia's constant reflux and desaturations. We had tried different reflux medicines, but nothing seemed to work. She still had many episodes of reflux daily.

"Next week," I said.

"Well, please keep me updated on what he says about her reflux." Her eyebrows furrowed as she handed Alessia back to me.

I imagined what it would be like to throw up every day like Alessia as I looked at her pale face. I could feel the tears coming in.

"Thank you, Dr. Squires, for everything." I grabbed the two car seats with my babies safely buckled and headed out the door. "Thank you, God, for sending such a fabulous pediatrician our way," I whispered.

## An Amazing Little Girl with Rhombencephalosynapsis

The days went by and Alessia kept desaturating and refluxing. I had already met several times with Dr. Pineiro, her GI doctor. He was from Puerto Rico, and I had lived in Puerto Rico for a few years when I was a child. My mother's ex-husband was a pilot and we got transferred to different cities all the time. We lived in Puerto Rico for two years when I was thirteen years old. I adapted well to Puerto Rico and learned a lot about the Puerto Rican culture. We had that cultural similarity that made Dr. Pineiro and I compatible. He was a polite and loving gastroenterologist. He was impressed at how well both babies grew, even if Alessia vomited constantly. "I think it would be a good idea to insert a jejunum tube through her PEG tube, to try to decrease her reflux," he said in one of her follow-up appointments. I could feel the sweat starting to drip from my forehead as my eyes widened. "Is this going to be another surgery?" I asked before he could finish the sentence.

"No, not at all!" he chuckled. "It's a quite simple procedure that can be done while she is awake. We just insert a very thin tube through her PEG tube all the way to her jejunum, which is a part of her intestines. This way, we bypass the stomach so the milk can go directly into her intestines. She will not have any milk in her stomach, so she won't have anything to vomit." The sincerity in his face made me trust him. It was clear that he cared about Alessia and was doing his best to try to help her. Without hesitation I agreed to the J-tube placement.

My mother wanted Ronaldo, Thiago, and me to have a family day without the girls. Ronaldo and I needed a break, and Thiago needed to have some one-to-one time with us. My mother came to my house to take care of the girls, and the three of us were headed to Lake Norman with my stepfather to ride on his boat.

Thiago's face beamed and his eyes sparkled. He couldn't contain his excitement when we told him he was going to ride a boat with his mom and dad . . . the three of us together like it had once been. The waters were calm, and it wasn't too hot—the perfect 70-degree temperature. Although I felt terrible about it, I enjoyed being on the boat without any medical duties. I called my mother frequently to check on the girls. "They're fine," my mother assured me.

I enjoyed the breeze caressing my face as the boat moved through the water. The relaxing tunes of Pure Moods played on the boat radio. Thiago sat on the edge of the boat trying to spot a fish or two. We anchored the boat and dove into the water like we were all little kids. The lake water so refreshing on my skin. We splashed and played with Thiago . . . the three of us together just like it had once been. Ronaldo and I drank beer and cracked some jokes with my stepfather. I even got tipsy since I hadn't drunk alcohol in a while. There was a beautiful sun setting on the horizon of the lake—pink, orange, and red. The water reflected the colors and was so tranquil. I felt guilty, for a moment, that my girls were not there to enjoy the sight. But that guilt quickly went away with how happy Thiago was to get his parents all to himself for a few hours. It's a difficult task to have all your children happy at one time.

"We should start to head back," my stepfather said, and we turned back to the dock. I missed my girls terribly, but I was also extremely thankful to have had the opportunity to spend quality time with my son and husband.

Back at home, my mother had it all under control. The girls were fed, bathed, and already put to sleep by the time we arrived. "Looks like you guys had fun!" She looked exhausted. She already had dark circles from a day with her granddaughters. She never once told me if it was hectic, though. For her it was a pleasure to take care of the girls for us to go out with Thiago.

I slept a solid three hours before Alessia woke up. I was back at my nursing job, and her color looked off again. I waited for the reflux to come, her oxygen levels desaturating. But she continued desaturating and didn't throw up. After a while, her oxygen level started to increase, but it never got back to the 90s. It lingered around the high 80s for the whole night. I lay next to her the whole night and stroked her back, stimulating her to breathe every time she would desaturate below 80. The pulse oximeter alarm went off constantly. "What is it, baby?" I asked, as if she could respond. I had a gut-wrenching feeling something was terribly wrong. Thank God the nurse will be here tomorrow to check on her, I thought, as I tried to comfort my anxiety. I did not get any more sleep that night.

Early the following morning the nurse came to check on Alessia. I told her about her desaturations throughout the night. Her eyes grew large, and her eyebrows furrowed as she looked at Alessia. "Her color is off," she nervously told me as she picked Alessia up.

"Yes, I'm worried. She has had this color since last night. What should I do?"

The nurse took her stethoscope out and listened to her lungs. She asked me to bring the pulse oximeter machine downstairs so she could check her oxygen levels. It was in the 70s and it was not coming back up. "You guys need to hurry to the hospital!" she exclaimed. Ronaldo and I were speechless. "Quickly, you need to take her in," she said again. We quickly jumped out of our chairs and grabbed Alessia, Sophia, and Thiago and drove nervously to Levine Children's Hospital. This was the first time we were heading to the emergency room, and we were panicked.

Ronaldo dropped me and Alessia off at the front door of the emergency room while he went to park and wait for my mother who was going to meet us at Levine to take Thiago and Sophia. I carried Alessia in her car seat in one hand and the pulse oximeter machine in the other hand as

I rushed through the front doors of the ER. As I was waiting in line to check in, I looked down at Alessia and her face was suddenly blue, and the pulse oximeter machine began alarming. "HELP!" I screamed. "She's blue! She isn't breathing, oh my God, please help me!"

The front desk receptionist looked at Alessia and I could see the fear in her eyes. She immediately brought us back to the ER. My heart was about to explode out of my chest from fear. My body started shaking and I started sobbing. "Oh my God!" I sobbed. "She is dying, SHE'S NOT BREATHING!" I cried at the top of my lungs, as I felt myself gasping for air. The emergency nurse rushed towards us and took Alessia out of her car seat. She started shaking her and strongly stroking her back to wake her up so she would breathe. Suddenly I heard a gasp of air. She was still alive!

The nurse rushed her to one of the rooms. Within five minutes, there were ten different people in Alessia's room. I looked at my daughter's lifeless body on the bed. She looked pale and still a little gray. I couldn't say anything. I was in shock. "Excuse me, Mrs. Costabel . . . excuse me," the ER doctor keep tapping me. "What are her medical conditions? When did she start turning blue? Did she throw up during the night? When was she discharged from the NICU?" The ER doctor kept asking me all sorts of questions, but all I could do was watch in horror as a team of medical personnel worked on Alessia's tiny body. One was putting an IV in, the other was suctioning saliva from her mouth, another was attaching the nasal oxygen cannula on her nose, another was undressing her, the other was monitoring the machines, the other was sticking the leads on her chest to monitor her heart rate and respiratory rate. I stood there unable to move during all this chaos as I watched my daughter fight for her life.

# An Amazing Little Girl with Rhombencephalosynapsis

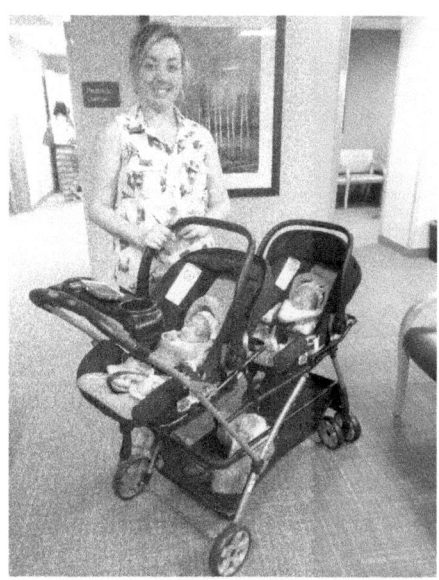

*Taking the girls to Alessia's doctor appointments, June 2015.
Photo Credit: Jaime Monslave*

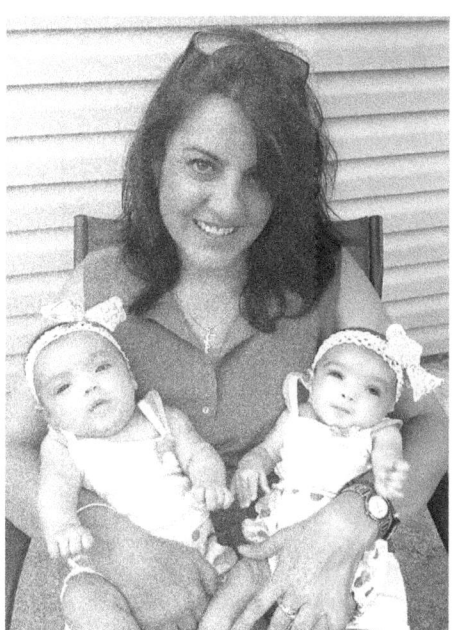

*My mom with the girls, July 2015.
Photo Credit: Stephanie Detjen Costabel*

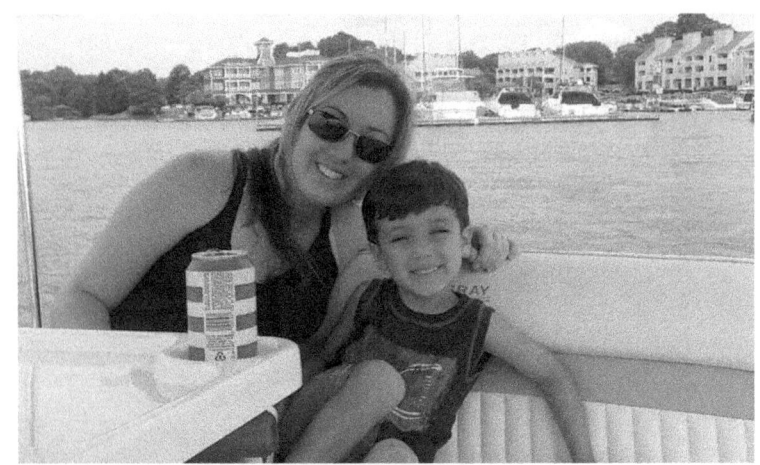

*Thiago and me at the lake, July 2015*
*Photo Credit: Ronaldo Cruz*

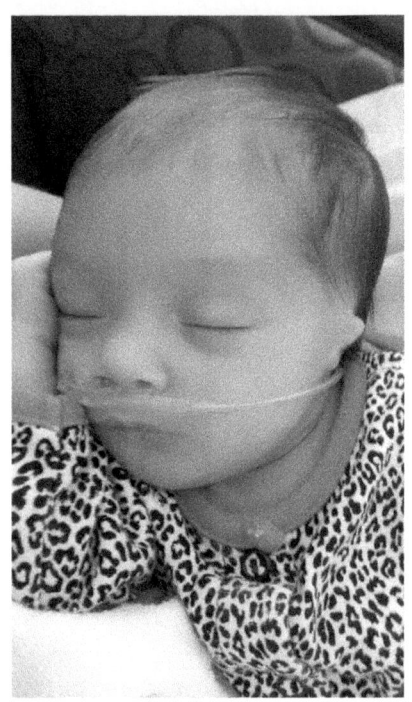

*Alessia Hospitalization, July 2015*
*Photo Credit: Stephanie Detjen Costabel*

# 9

Apnea of prematurity, the doctors confirmed after a couple of days of studying her desaturations as an admitted patient at the hospital. Dr. Pineiro had been called and they decided they were going to insert the J tube while she was inpatient. They thought that part of her desaturations was due to aspirating her reflux. It was a rather simple procedure to switch from a G tube to a J tube. A skinny tube was carefully inserted through her PEG tube and slowly pushed down to reach her jejunum. With the help of an X-ray machine, they could verify the exact placement of the J tube.

With the placement of the J tube came less reflux because she was fed directly into her intestines so there was not much in her stomach for her to vomit. Unfortunately, she was still desaturating her oxygen levels. She required one liter of oxygen while she slept for her not to desaturate her oxygen levels below 80.

Pulmonology was called. They ordered a sleep study to see how bad her apnea got while she slept. They didn't do sleep studies on babies at Levine Children's Hospital at the time, so we had to schedule an overnight sleep study at UNC Chapel Hill Sleep Clinic. The first available was two months from then, unfortunately, so the plan was to send her home with oxygen for when she slept at night until we could have the sleep study.

She was also prescribed caffeine to stimulate her lungs to breathe.

Inpatient was nothing like the NICU. The children had their own rooms and one nurse had to care for more than one child. You could sleep with your child in their own room, but as the nurses often came in throughout the night to check on the baby's vital signs, Alessia would wake up and then take hours to fall back asleep again. I missed being at home with Thiago and Sophia, but the five days at the hospital gave me a lot of time to research what was happening to Alessia. I had a gut-wrenching feeling the doctors were wrong and that the apnea was due to something else. The more I inquired on the RES Facebook page, the more concerned I became about another potential problem Alessia might have.

Many children with RES had Chiari, and the symptoms were quite like what Alessia was experiencing. Alessia was discharged from the NICU without oxygen, and yet one month later she needed oxygen to live. I had mentioned that to her doctors many times, but they were not able to see Chiari in her CT scans. But since RES is an exceedingly rare brain malformation, they hadn't seen a child with RES before. I learned from the Facebook group that Chiari was tricky to diagnose. There were a few moms in the group that had to push for a particular MRI called a flexion extension MRI, which was a sophisticated type of MRI unavailable at Levine. I probably could have pushed for an order to have a flex extension MRI at UNC Chapel Hill, but since her CT scans looked normal and the doctors assured me that she did not have Chiari, I let it go.

When we were discharged, we went home with an oxygen tank, as well as another medicine prescription for caffeine. The list of medical supplies was growing, instead of decreasing. The following few days after she was discharged were rough. She was restless and cried constantly. I started to think that the caffeine was making her irritable. Her cheeks were raw from the stickers that kept her nasal cannula in place at night. The reflux had decreased since the J tube, but she would still throw up her secretions that accumulated in her throat, as well as stomach acids.

I was at a loss as how to help her and cried watching her be so uncomfortable.

When I called the pulmonology and GI doctors, they kept saying to give it time—that she would eventually be taken off of the caffeine and oxygen because it was just apnea of prematurity, and she would eventually grow out of it. Deep down inside I knew that it was not just apnea of prematurity.

Weeks went by and we just learned how to deal with it. By September, I was a pro at working the oxygen machines and the nasal cannula. The follow-ups with the rest of the specialists including ENT and Audiology continued.

Then one warm, September day I received a phone call.

"Hi, Mrs. Costabel, it's Novant Audiology. We wanted to let you know that Alessia's BAHA (bone anchored hearing aid) has arrived." I had called about fifty times that month to check on the status of the order.

My smile widened from ear-to-ear as I started jumping up and down from the joy. "Fabulous!" I exclaimed. "When can we come pick it up?" I asked.

"You're more than welcome to come later today if you would like," the audiologist replied.

I immediately called Ronaldo and told him the great news. He came home early from work, and we headed to Audiology with Sophia, Thiago, and Alessia. It was going to be the first time my daughter would hear my voice . . . five months after she was born.

I dressed both girls in beautiful green summer dresses with matching headbands. I loved dressing them alike for outings. Everywhere we went I would hear the "Oohs" and "Aww . . . twins!" from complete strangers. The only thing that differentiated the girls was Alessia's tiny ear and her feeding tube bag. The size difference wasn't too noticeable. Alessia's color was always pale compared to her sister and she was much skinnier than Sophia, but at first glance nobody could tell the difference. Especially since they were always dressed alike.

At the Audiology Clinic, Alessia's bone anchored hearing device was waiting for her. The BAHA is a hearing aid that is attached to a soft band that goes around the head like a headband. Sound is picked up by the processor and travels through the skull to the cochlea. It's different from a cochlear implant because it isn't implanted into the skin and the sound travels through bone. With a cochlear implant, sound travels through a wire into the cochlea that is surgically placed in the ear. Cochlear implants are for sensorineural hearing loss while a BAHA is for conductive hearing loss.

I had my camera ready to take a video of Alessia hearing for the first time. The audiologist unwrapped the hearing aid processor, put the batteries in, and turned it on. They snapped it on to the soft band and placed it over her head and waited until the beeping stopped. It was on now and she could hear. "Holaaaaaa Alessiaaaa!" we all said at the same time, like we were greeting our baby for the first time. She suddenly froze, furrowing her eyebrows. She held her breath, looked at the audiologist first, then to Ronaldo, and then to me. She then gave us the biggest smile we had ever seen from her. I started crying from the joy. She was hearing our voices for the first time in her life, and it made her so happy.

"What is that?" the audiologist asked her in a cute baby voice. "Is that Mommy?" Alessia looked towards me. Everyone shed a tear in that room. Nobody could hold back their emotions watching the amazing expression she made when hearing for the first time.

She put on a proud face as we all cheered her on. She knew she was being watched. She also knew we were all excited for her. That was the first time I knew she understood her surroundings and that she was incredibly smart.

The following days, Alessia was discovering new sounds with her hearing aid. She was obsessed with a snowman stuffed animal toy that would sing "Frosty the Snowman" every time you pressed its hand. No matter what she was doing, as soon as that toy started singing, she would pause to look at it, intrigued by the melody. She also showed interest in the "Itsy-Bitsy Spider" song . . . Her hearing therapist that came to our house once a week was incredibly surprised at how well she was able to locate sound. I was warned by the audiologist that she might be more irritable as she got used to all the sounds, and we might have to take the BAHA off throughout the day. She would indeed pull the BAHA off many times throughout the day.

But more than irritability, it seemed as if the BAHA was causing headaches. I wasn't able to tell for sure if it was headaches until she started sitting unassisted at approximately eight months old. That's when she seemed to have her head slumped to the side when she had her BAHA on.

The following months, we worked with her feeding therapist on swallowing, and with her hearing therapist on locating sounds. Physical therapy would work with her and help her learn to crawl and sit unassisted. Occupational therapy would work on play therapy and teach her how to use certain toys appropriately for her age. She was still on oxygen at night but was able to be weaned from one liter to half a liter. We were able to successfully wean her off the caffeine as well.

But the one thing that never improved was her reflux.

Even with a J tube, she would still throw up bile, secretions, stomach acids . . . It wasn't a whole lot since she didn't have any formula in her stomach, but it still was enough to make her extremely uncomfortable. The reflux caught up to her eventually and she ended up developing a cough that was unbearable to hear—as if she was coughing her brains out.

It turned out to be aspiration pneumonia. The days went by, and the albuterol prescribed wasn't helping, nor the antibiotics. There wasn't anything I could do except comfort her every time she had a coughing spell. She would cough so much she would throw up. The secretions and stomach acids would get into her nasal cannula, and then she would breathe in her own secretions and throw up again. I would change her nasal cannula, her clothes, and sheets multiple times during the night. "Please, God! Please stop this coughing!" I would scream out at the top of the top of my lungs as I kneeled, begging for help. She was in so much pain and so uncomfortable. She would turn gray and gasp for air while she was drowning in her own throw up. I would cry in agony, not knowing how to help her. I was in hell watching my daughter slowly and painfully dying. She was not getting better, no matter how much albuterol and prednisone I gave her.

Finally, her Pulmonology and GI team decided she needed a Nissen fundoplication, which is a surgery in which they would tie the top of her stomach so she would not throw up anymore. They thought she would never get better unless she stopped vomiting and aspirating her stomach acids and secretions. We were all trying to avoid a tracheostomy placement. With the Nissen fundoplication she would still be able to swallow but would be unable to throw up. Or at least not as much.

Her surgery was scheduled early in the morning, February 26. She wasn't even a year old and was already having her second surgery. The roofs of the houses were covered in frost. My mother went with me so I would not be by myself throughout the procedure, while Ronaldo stayed at home with Thiago and Sophia. Alessia was still coughing and hadn't fully recovered from her pneumonia yet. Her lungs still had fluid in them, but the benefits outweighed the risks of her having surgery while she was so sick. I was terrified. My mother was scared. Everyone was scared. We hadn't slept in days just agonizing over this procedure. I prayed so hard. I was so sick to my stomach that by the time she went back to the OR, I had already gone to the bathroom five times. The pre-op nurse checked all Alessia's vital signs, and we spoke to the doctors. We went over the procedure and the OR was ready for her. Anesthesia wanted to keep her intubated after the surgery because of how sick her lungs were. I kissed her cheek and said one final goodbye before she was taken back. My mother and I could not hold back our tears. Two mothers in the same room, each one worried about their daughter. The nurses felt sorry for us and kept assuring us that everything was going to be okay. The hours we spent in the OR waiting room were nerve-wracking. I paced from one side of the room to the other nervously waiting for the procedure to be finished. After about three hours, I had no more nails left to bite.

"Alessia Cruz," the waiting room receptionist called out. My mother and I rushed to the front desk. "She is finished with the procedure. The doctor will come out and talk to you guys," she said as she guided us to the conference room. We sat in that conference room and waited. Thoughts of bad news or that something did not go as planned were all I could think of while we waited. I had been in that room before—there were three comfortable sofas facing a large window that overlooked uptown Charlotte. The sun reflected off the building windows, making for a breathtaking view. There were drawings made by children that had received care at Levine hanging on the walls. Pastel colors, I thought. A way to relax you before you get the bad news. It was hard for me to think positively while Alessia was so sick.

The doctor finally walked in after what seemed like an hour. "She did well," he said with a charming smile. "She has a pretty big stomach, so I was able to wrap the top portion of it rather tightly." He made a simulation with his fingers to demonstrate how he wrapped the top of her stomach. "We are going to keep her intubated and transfer her to PICU for a few days. We want to make sure her lungs show improvement before extubating her. But overall, everything went as expected. You can go see her here in a few minutes once she is transferred."

I let out a huge sigh of relief, and tears started rolling down my cheeks. "Thank you so much! I was so worried that she wouldn't go through it well." I wanted to hug him. All that worrying I'd done, and she did so well.

Back at the PICU, Alessia looked so fragile lying in her crib, intubated, and completely sedated. She had four small bandages on her incisions. The one above her belly button was the shape of a heart. That's cute, I thought. The PICU nurse greeted us and saw I was looking at the heart-shaped bandage. "Dr. Cramer always does that with all of his patients, like a trademark," she said as she giggled.

"That's sweet he would take out the time to cut out a little heart on the bandage." I stroked Alessia's hair.

After a few days in the PICU, she was ready to be extubated. She was breathing over the ventilator and the doctors were confident that she would be able to breathe on her own. Extubating is an exciting step up in the PICU. It's the last step before being transferred to the regular pediatric floor. For this procedure, the room is filled with many different specialists: nurses, the doctors, respiratory therapists . . . You can feel the nervousness and adrenaline throughout the entire room.

Alessia was successfully extubated and transferred to the pediatric floor. The following step was to make sure she tolerated her feeds. After a few days in the regular pediatric floor, she was able to tolerate continuous feeds and was not vomiting anymore. Success!

She was discharged from Levine Children's Hospital after six days. We were all ecstatic to have her back home. I was particularly happy that she wouldn't throw up as often as she had been.

No more surgeries, I thought. Hopefully not throwing up and not aspirating would head towards improvement in her medical health. As I lay myself to sleep that first night at home, I couldn't help but feel butterflies seeing how cute she was. She was a beauty indeed.

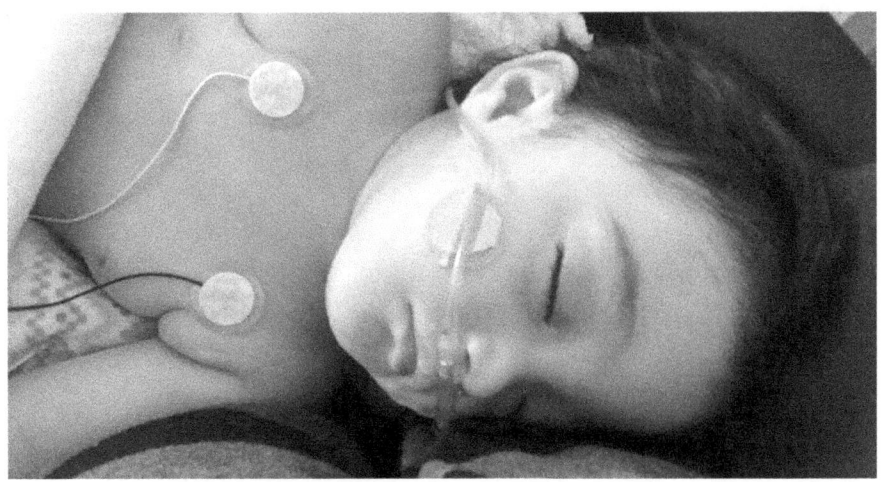

*Alessia at her Nissen Fundoplication Surgery, February 2016*
*Photo Credit: Stephanie Deitjen Costable*

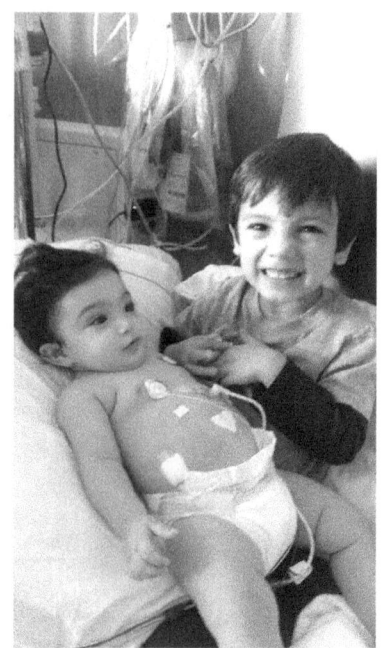
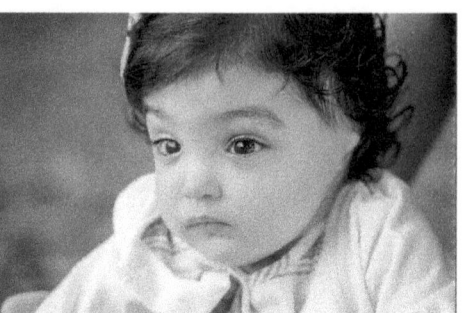
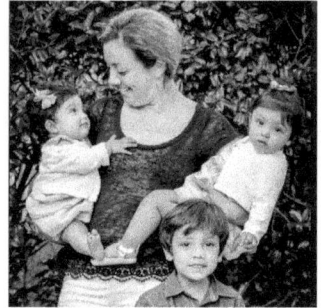

*Thiago with Alessia after her Nissen Fundoplication Surgery, February 2016*
*Photo credit: Stephanie Detjen Costabel*

*Levine's NICU reunion, 2016*
*Photo Credit: Flashes of Hope*

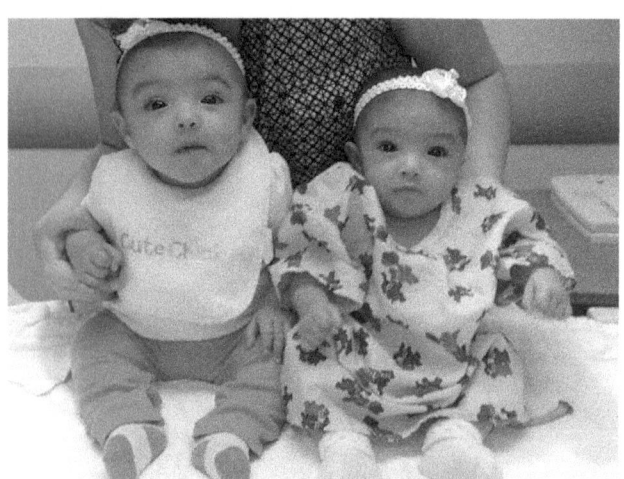

*Sophia accompanying Alessia to her J-tube placement, 2015*
*Photo credit: Stephanie Detjen Costabel*

# 10

It was a special day. My girls were turning one.

I had planned a huge first birthday party for the girls. It was a miracle they had made it alive to their first birthday, so I went all out. I invited close to fifty people to a beautiful venue on Lake Norman. We got there two hours early to decorate the clubhouse for the guests. I decorated eight round tables with white tablecloths and pink flower centerpieces my mother had made. I was obsessed with baby owls, so I had ordered small owl candles for souvenirs that I placed neatly around the centerpieces on each table. There were large pink and white balloons covering the ceiling of the clubhouse. A friend of mine had volunteered to fill up the balloons and help decorate. A collage that I had been working on for over two months hung gracefully from the cake table. Each picture of the girls reflected their first year on this Earth. I even handmade the happy birthday sign in pastel pink and purple colors large enough to extend over the large windows overlooking the lake. By the time we were done, the whole place looked like a masterpiece of art.

The sky was turquoise blue without a single cloud visible. The fresh spring breeze caressed my cheeks and rays of sun beamed through the tall trees. The water of the lake was calm as it reflected the sun like a mirror.

I had planned that birthday party for over two months. I even had a DJ to entertain the guests. The MoMo twin pregnancy, my inpatient stay, the NICU stage, Alessia's surgeries—there was so much to celebrate. We had gone through all of this in one year and all of us made it out in one piece.

I invited all of Alessia's doctors and therapists. I wanted them to be a part of the celebration. But only my dear friend Dr. Squires came to the birthday, out of all Alessia's specialists. It was an act of kindness from her part that spoke so highly of her. She was genuine and I deeply appreciated her presence.

All our family and friends that we invited attended. They all were amazed at Alessia's progress and how we'd overcome our difficult year. The children played with the bubble machine that I had rented. Sophia was already learning how to walk so she was all over the place. Both girls dressed in white onesies with a pink tutu. I had gotten matching headbands with huge flowers. Alessia was able to sit unassisted, but unable to bear weight on her legs yet to stand, so she was content in her stroller. Thiago had fun playing in the forest around the lake with the other children of the party. The adults socialized, eating appetizers and sipping on champagne.

Everyone watched with joy as Sophia tasted the icing from their cake on her fingers. Alessia was not particularly amused by the texture of the cake, and she never put any icing in her mouth, but she was entertained trying to wipe the icing off her hands. I was able to capture a photo of a tender moment when Alessia looked at my mother who was kneeling next to her and gave her the prettiest appreciative smile when my mom wiped her hands. The sky filled with orange and yellow as the sun settled over the horizon. We took amazing photos of the family with that beautiful sunset. It was a birthday party I will forever cherish.

Alessia had been somewhat stable those few months after her Nissen fundoplication. She was still on oxygen at night, and rather fussy during the day. She had developed a corneal ulcer on her left eye that was not healing as fast as the ophthalmologist wanted. Eye problems are common in the RES world. Trigeminal anesthesia often goes hand in hand with Rhombencephalosynapsis. Alessia lacked sensation in her corneas, so picking at them was one of her favorite hobbies. The decreased blink reflex would cause her to get multiple abrasions. The eye could not protect itself from the environment because she didn't blink as often as a normal child would. She touched her eyes a great deal, and before she turned one, she already had a central corneal scar. We saw ophthalmology weekly in Charlotte. When they were out of options to improve the corneal healing process, they referred us to the Duke Eye Center in Durham. After an amniotic membrane graft and a bandage contact lens, Alessia's ulcer finally healed, but it did leave a significant central scar. It was the first of many ulcers she would have and the beginning of the deterioration of her vision.

The Nissen fundoplication and J tube had stopped Alessia's reflux for a few months. But by the summer, Alessia was gagging on her own secretions.

We had another swallow study—her swallow was not getting any better. She couldn't manage her own secretions. She wasn't aspirating as much as before, but she was still aspirating some of her own secretions. She had a persistent cough. It was the way her body protected her airway from aspirating, but her cough wasn't strong enough to provide full protection. Yet it was encouraging that she could cough. Pulmonology was convinced that if she stopped coughing, she would eventually need a tracheostomy to suction out her secretions.

The sleep study they had ordered a few months ago was finally scheduled for a couple of weeks after her first birthday.

Alessia and I left our house at 5 p.m. to be in Raleigh at the check-in time at 7 p.m. The highway was busy from afternoon traffic. It was a two-hour drive, and Jatrin, who lived in Raleigh, was going to meet me at the clinic to help us settle in. Alessia had been calm throughout the car ride, which was not common for her, but I didn't mind it at all. I was just hoping she wouldn't fall asleep because then it would be hard for her to sleep during the sleep study. We arrived at UNC Chapel Hill and checked in. We were guided to our sleep room. The room looked like a hotel room—there was a comfortable looking queen-sized bed with a crib next to it. There was a plasma TV hanging on the wall as well as a private bathroom that contained toothbrush, toothpaste, hand soap, towels, etc.

Not bad, I thought. I was exhausted from the drive so I hoped I would get some sleep, although I knew it would be hard. The sleep technician walked in with a friendly sparkle in her eyes. "What a beautiful child!" she said, as she handed over a clipboard with the forms I needed to fill out. She had a warm personality and a comforting tone to her voice. I wasn't particularly worried about the sleep study, just a bit anxious as to what to expect.

"So how does this work?" I asked.

"Girl. You look terrified!" she giggled. "It's not bad. I will attach a lot of different probes all over her head and body to monitor her brain activity while she sleeps. There are many probes, so it will take a while to get all of them on. But you guys should be all set for the night around 9 p.m. The sleep study is over at 6 a.m." I nodded as I texted my sister letting her know what room we were in.

"My sister is out front, could you let the front desk know, so they can guide her here, please?" The technician nodded and left.

Ten minutes later Jatrin arrived. "Holy shit, this room is far," she said, wiping the sweat from her forehead. "Sorry I'm late." She is a registered nurse, so she already knew a lot about sleep studies and medical terminology. She lived in the area so always tried to go with me to UNC or

Duke for Alessia's appointments.

We hurried to bathe Alessia and tried to get her tired so she would sleep while they attached all her probes. Then I gave Alessia her meds and started her feeds again. Right at 8 p.m. the technician came back with a cart full of wires and machines. The technician carefully stuck each probe on her head using a sticky wax that would keep it in place. My sister and I watched with awe.

By 9 p.m. the last probe was attached. There were at least fifty wires coming from Alessia's head, and another twenty from her chest and back.

The technician slipped a headwrap on and secured all the wires to one side. Miraculously, Alessia slept through it all and my sister and I were amazed. "How in the world is it possible she could actually fall asleep with so many wires and probes connected to her?" My sister and I looked at each other in disbelief.

Alessia slept undisturbed until approximately 3 a.m. She then started wiggling around and soon woke up and realized what she had on her head. She started messing with the wires and pulling at them. They were able to record six straight hours of sleep, which was the minimum they needed to complete the sleep study. After 4 a.m., the technician realized she wasn't going to go back to sleep, so she ended the sleep study and came into the room to remove the probes. That lasted about an hour, and by 5:30 a.m. we were in the van heading back to Charlotte. Alessia's hair looked like she had been swimming in glue. Her face was covered in the sticker residue that had kept her nasal cannula in place during the sleep study. I felt like I needed toothpicks to keep my eyelids opened. I was beyond tired. We got home at 7:30 a.m. and I didn't say good morning to anyone. I handed over Alessia to Ronaldo and passed out on the living room couch.

The sleep study results took about a week to come through to our pulmonologist.

Pulmonology called me to let me know that the results were too complex to discuss over the phone. They needed to see me in person. They scheduled me four days after they called. My sense of worry was heightened throughout those four days of waiting. I wondered what could be so complex that they couldn't discuss over the phone.

The RES Facebook page proved to be the greatest source of information about Rhombencephalosynapsis and its comorbidities. Anytime I was worried or had a question, I posted in the group and always got helpful answers. So, when I posted about Alessia's multiple difficulties and now the sleep study, one mom replied with a great deal of information. Deanna Jones truly opened my eyes to a world I didn't know existed. As I read her reply, suddenly everything made sense.

*Oh my gosh. Chiari. It was our undiagnosed nightmare for years and we literally talked to doctors across the country, trying to get help and get it figured out. Not even Doherty's lab could help. Please, have the girl checked for a Chiari. This will be long, but it needs some explanation.*

*Chiari is a gray area in neurosurgery. They've only been operating on them for like 30 years or so, and the jury is out on when to intervene. It's a controversial topic in neurosurgical topics. You'll have surgeons that adamantly disagree with each other. Just because there is one, doesn't mean it needs intervention. It depends on how symptomatic the kid is, and different neurosurgeons will define "symptomatic" differently. A Chiari is just when the cerebellum is herniated or protruding through the hole at the base of the skull. Old school neurosurgery says you intervene when there is no fluid flow between the cerebellum and the brain stem and there is a syrinx. Others will look at other indicators, like if there is fluid flow on the opposite side of the cerebellum toward the back of the skull, how steep the angle of the tentorium is, if there is a little notch on the brainstem indicating tightness, etc. A lot of Chiari symptoms overlap with issues that rhombencephalosynapsis can cause, so surgeons will say the kid has a malformed cerebellum so of COURSE they are going to have symptoms of a dysfunctional cerebellum.*

*It is really an uphill battle for our babies to prove they would benefit from surgery. If the kid has a Chiari and has symptoms of a Chiari that overlap symptoms of rhombencephalosynapsis, but the Chiari isn't definitively too tight, you have to have them do a flexion extension MRI of the cervical spine. Basically, when they do an MRI for a child, they tip the child's head back to keep the airway open. That position, lying down, messes up how a Chiari looks because it allows gravity to pull the cerebellum back up into the skull a little bit, so the herniation isn't as far. It may open up a slightly wider area of cerebral spinal fluid flow than if the kid would have sat up, and really just makes a Chiari look better than it really is. A flexion extension MRI is different in that they scan the child in that position, but then they move the head into a neutral position and scan, and then tip the head forward and scan. That gives them a better picture of how the Chiari is behaving than just a regular, tipped back MRI. Our kids' cerebellums are smaller than normal so they also can "slip."*

*Oh my gosh, this was a nightmare for us. My son's Chiari looked like it shouldn't be symptomatic because he had great fluid flow in the front, and he did not have a syrinx. It wasn't until someone tipped his head forward on an MRI that we could see how drastically it kinked his brainstem in that position. He totally lost his ability to eat and drink orally before someone figured it out. Everyone kept saying it was rhombencephalosynapsis and kids with RES don't swallow anyway. Which is total BS. Plus, he had GRADUATED FROM FEEDING THERAPY. It was a loss of skills. That Chiari that looked great with a regular MRI was ugly when they got in there. His tonsils were herniated so tight they were white from lack of blood flow. He had a bunch of membranes locking it into place that had to be cleaned up, and one of his cerebellar tonsils had been compressing the other one so tightly that it was atrophic.*

*Right before the surgery, my non-aspirator was completely coughing and gagging and choking on reflux. He was barfing like crazy, had unreal headaches, urine retention problems, and horrific apneic/desaturation episodes that were NOT consistent from night to night. Supposedly that doesn't happen either. Disordered sleep is supposed to be consistent from night to night. When we decompressed him, it all got better? Like, within days. It was absolutely his Chiari.*

*If you have a neurologist or a neurosurgeon who is approachable and willing to look at it differently because your kid's cerebellum is shaped differently, you're golden. Push for a flexion extension MRI of the cervical spine to distinguish if it's RES causing problems or if it is the Chiari causing problems. If we hadn't done the flex/extension, we never would have seen how bad my son's Chiari was messing with his brainstem.*

I put my phone down and suddenly I was in survival mode, my heart racing realizing what I was up against. I had to get her doctors to listen to me, there was no doubt about it. Alessia definitely had Chiari. My hope was that the pulmonologist would listen to me, especially now that he saw something very concerning in her sleep study results.

The day finally arrived to go over Alessia's sleep study results. I picked out a professional outfit and did my hair and makeup. Maybe if I looked professional, they would take my concerns more seriously, I thought. I was incredibly naïve back then.

Alessia's pulmonologist was a charming, older man who had some experience with Chiari malformation. You could tell he loved kids by the way he would play with Alessia every time we had an appointment with him. He always had admiration for her big brown eyes.

"We have a lot to talk about." He smiled as he shut the door behind him. I gulped as he continued. "Alessia had 104 events during her sleep study. She had 10 obstructive, 10 mixed, 22 central, and 62 hypopneas. The lowest she desaturated to was 80 before she would bring herself back up again."

"So, what does this all mean?" I asked nervously.

"She has to continue on a half liter of oxygen during sleep. She hasn't outgrown her apnea of prematurity," he said, handing me the sleep study results.

I started feeling the fumes coming out of my ears, and I shook my head. "We need to get her evaluated for Chiari malformation." I got up from the chair. "She is gagging. She is coughing. She is aspirating. She still has bouts of reflux here and there and now this sleep study results. The central component of her apnea has to come from her brain. She has a Chiari. I am sure of it."

He stared at me, intrigued. I started showing him the posts on the RES Facebook page of the examples of other kids that had RES and Chiari not shown on regular MRI scans. I had memorized Deanna's Facebook reply and explained why Alessia needed a flexion extension MRI. I was talking fast and I'm sure I sounded desperate.

I'd read about a little girl with RES and Chiari who had died due to her apnea. They hadn't gotten her Chiari decompressed in time. She died in her sleep from brainstem compression. I feared the same would happen to Alessia. I convinced the doctor to at least offer to call the neurologist and ask about the possibility of a flex extension MRI. He was impressed by my knowledge and agreed with Chiari being a possibility. I left the appointment content and relieved someone had heard me and was actually going to try and do something about it.

That night I felt relief as I lay down for the night. I hope he actually does call the neurologist, I thought as I drifted off to sleep.

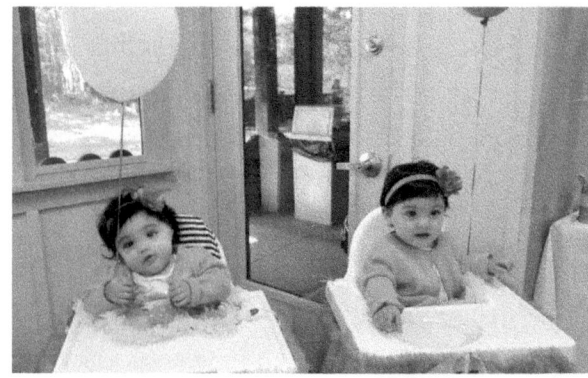

*Sophia and Alessia at their first birthday, April 2016*
*Photo Credit:*
*Stephanie Detjen Costabel*

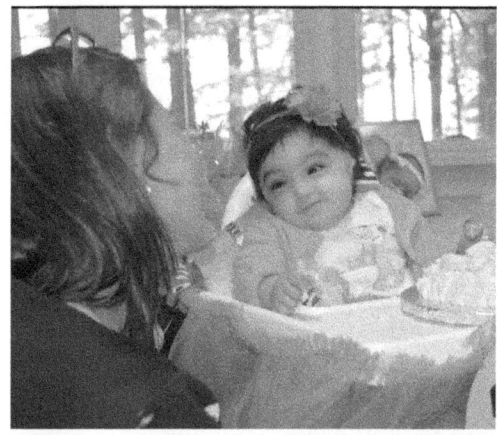

*My Mom and Alessia at her first birthday, April 2016*
*Photo Credit:*
*Stephanie Detjen Costabel*

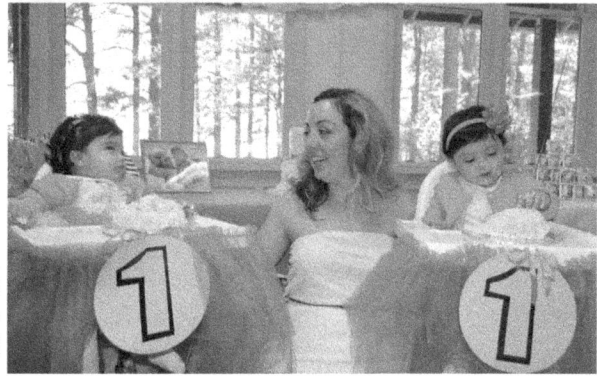

*The girls' first birthday party, April 2016*
*Photo Credit:*
*Stephanie Detjen Costabel*

## 11

Two weeks went by and there was still no call from neurology. I was losing my patience and Alessia was not getting better.

Alessia was not making any gains with the feeding therapist that came to the house, and there were more options at an actual clinic, so we had started feeding therapy at a feeding clinic that specialized in feeding and speech therapy for special-needs children. The feeding therapist was a sweet lady who had firsthand experience with parenting a child with feeding difficulties. She had adopted a little girl with special needs who had trouble swallowing. This helped me emotionally, because she understood what it means to be the mom of the child you are trying to help. She tried everything. She started with vital stim to help with her swallowing muscles. She would attach electric probes to Alessia's neck to stimulate the throat muscles to work in coordination with each other and swallow safely. After a couple of months, we realized that it wasn't really working. The therapist proceeded with a behavioral approach to feeding. She was training Alessia to open her mouth every time a dry spoon was offered. Alessia would get a reward every time she opened her mouth, whether it was a light-up toy, sparkly beads (which she had obsession with), or something else that grabbed her attention.

I noticed that feeding therapy was hard on Alessia. She hated opening her mouth up to accept the spoon. She was learning to open her mouth and accept the spoon because she wanted the reward, not because she was hungry or even liked the taste of certain foods. I understood it was the start of having an eating routine. But for a child who partially aspirated when she swallowed, swallowing was painful for her, and she was terrified. I wholeheartedly disagreed with the behavioral approach to feeding therapy. Just think of how you would feel if you were trained to open up your mouth every time a spoon is offered, not because you are hungry or want to taste some food, but just because your duty is to open your mouth and accept a spoon. *I will give you what you want if you open your mouth* was what my daughter was learning. I didn't like that approach but knew the feeding therapist was trying everything in her power to get Alessia to eat.

I mentioned to the therapist about the possibility of Chiari malformation. She worked with Alessia's neurologist at the time. I explained to her that we could not proceed with feeding therapy if Alessia had Chiari malformation. She agreed it could be a possibility. "You must be persistent," the feeding therapist said one day. "You call Dr. Harper and demand to talk to her. Explain to the assistant that you need Dr. Harper to call you." I nodded. That was the most useful piece of advice I would ever receive, and I learned from it. Persistence on my part with Alessia's medical team is what has kept her alive. You must push the doctors to answer your questions, even if it takes fifty phone calls.

That afternoon, I called neurology and demanded to talk to Dr. Harper. I told the receptionist that if the neurologist did not think Chiari could be the explanation to her decline in health, then I needed her to call me and discuss as soon as possible.

After two days she finally called. "Hi, Mrs. Costabel. It's Dr. Harper, Alessia's neurologist, how are you?" she asked.

"Super relieved you have called," I said with a not-so-happy tone in my voice.

## An Amazing Little Girl with Rhombencephalosynapsis

"I have gotten your messages about your concern for Arnold Chiari Malformation for your daughter. Unfortunately, the specific MRI that you would like to have performed on Alessia is not offered here at Levine, but I did call neurosurgery and there is another MRI called a Chiari protocol MRI that we can schedule to check for Chiari. Basically, they will scan her cervical spine to look for evidence of Chiari. It goes together with a CINE—a specific MRI study to observe the flow of cerebrospinal fluid in the cervical region. This will show us if she indeed has Chiari and how severe it is."

I let out a sigh of relief. "Oh, thank God! I thought I was going to have to argue and fight to prove she has Chiari," I replied.

"I'm sorry it has taken a while to get back to you. I am actually moving to Virginia so I have been extremely busy leaving all of my patient's files to another neurologist, who will be taking over my caseload of patients." My heart sank. I had only met with Dr. Harper twice, but she seemed to be an understanding and knowledgeable neurologist, although hard to get a hold of for sure. I remember the Pediatric Care Team had called her many times when Alessia was inpatient but had a hard time reaching her. She had never considered Chiari to be a possibility, since her scans did not show her cerebellum protruding through her spinal canal. Now we would have to get used to another neurologist.

"Well, congratulations on your new job," I said, trying to sound enthusiastic. "I just hope whoever has Alessia's case will understand her complexities."

"I will make sure they do understand them," she said. "Dr. Grayer will be your neurologist from now on."

I remembered him. "Oh okay—I think I met him once in the NICU." He had been the on-call neurologist that had called me to discuss Alessia's first MRI results in the NICU. "I'll go ahead and schedule that MRI and then Dr. Grayer will call you to go over the results," Dr. Harper said.

"Thank you so much. Good luck in Virginia." My voice trembled as I hung up the phone.

June 29, 2016: Alessia was getting a Chiari protocol MRI, cerebral spinal fluid flow study, and ABR hearing test. I had read about low frequency hearing loss being a common symptom of Chiari malformation, so I pushed for that study to be included in her list of studies for that day. I wanted to make sure every corner was turned.

She was scheduled for 10 a.m. I was already used to the process: nothing to eat or drink past midnight, a.m. meds were okay to give, etc., etc.

I left Thiago and Sophia with Ronaldo, and we headed to Levine's at 8 a.m. We always had to be there two hours prior to the procedure time. Radiology was where we were headed, which had a more relaxed feeling than the OR. The fact she wasn't going to have to be operated on was reason enough for me to be calmer.

I checked in and filled out all the pre-op anesthesia forms. I always get nervous before Alessia has to go under anesthesia. My body trembles. My brain can't stop worrying. A full intubation with a child that has airway difficulties always has complications. Thankfully it was only an LMA (Laryngeal Mask Airway), so it was not a full airway intubation. She always did better with an LMA versus a full airway intubation. When it was time to let her go, I kissed her cheeks goodbye and said a little prayer, like always. "See you soon my sweet Alessia…" I whispered in her tiny ear as a tear fell down my cheek. It always hurts when I have to hand her over to somebody else's care. Once again, I was led to the waiting room. This time it would be five hours before I was able to see my daughter again.

I wasn't worried or nervous when I arrived in the waiting room. Even after she was done with the procedure, I would have to wait a few days before I got the results. The whole series of studies did take an extremely long time. It was close to four in the afternoon before she was out of the MRI room. They must have gotten scans of absolutely everything. I was glad. After an hour in recovery, she was ready to go home.

It had been a long day for Alessia and me. That night we both fell asleep before 8 p.m.

I was thankful she finally got the test for Chiari. Hopefully, I thought, she does have Chiari and it will eventually be decompressed, and her health will start to improve. It had been more than a year that I'd been dealing with Alessia's reflux, irritability, swallowing difficulties, apnea, oxygen use, aspiration pneumonias, etc. I needed an answer to explain her problems, and RES was not the only one. So many children had RES and could eat orally and live normally without so many obstacles. I wanted Alessia to get better.

The results of her studies took a couple of days. The wait was nerve-wracking. Her physical behaviors showed us her head was hurting—she would do these headstands while she was trying to learn how to crawl. She wasn't responding to sound the way she had responded before. She would get dizzy easily and lose her balance. Oxygen was still needed at night and even then, she was still desaturating her oxygen levels. She still gagged and coughed while trying to manage her secretions. She had left the NICU without oxygen and now she needed oxygen to live . . . or maybe she always needed it, but we didn't realize it until a month later when she turned gray.

It was an early summer morning, and I wasn't expecting a phone call from the neurologist so early. "Hi, Mrs. Costabel. It's Dr. Grayer." I let out a sigh of relief as my heart started racing while I listened.

"Hi, Dr. Grayer, I appreciate your call, I have waited for this call for a few days now and am so relieved my phone rang and it's you!" I said while my voice trembled.

"Yes, I am sure you have been anticipating this call. The results are in. She has a very mild Chiari malformation. It's very mild. I don't think she needs surgical intervention. Either way, I will put a referral out to neurosurgery for their opinion. Her ventricles are slightly enlarged, but not too concerning. Let's get neurosurgery's opinion on her Chiari, but just so you know, I don't think they are going to intervene." His tone was confident.

He continued, "Also, her middle ear is extremely malformed. The ABR hearing test shows a low-frequency hearing loss in her microtia ear, which has declined from her ABR results back from in the NICU. I have sent these new ABR results to her audiologist. They might need to change the settings of her hearing aid so she can hear better." Suddenly my vision became blurry. It was the results that I had anticipated, but I felt irritated that the neurologist had said it was a "mild" Chiari. I wondered if I would have to argue with neurosurgery to get them to intervene surgically. I remembered what the other moms had replied to my post on the RES page back when I inquired about Chiari. It would be a battle to get neurosurgery to intervene.

"Well, let's just wait and see what neurosurgery says . . . I have put the referral in so they should be contacting you soon."

What if her Chiari had been addressed earlier? Could we have avoided unnecessary surgeries? I asked myself this time and time again. Maybe she would be eating orally and not aspirating; maybe we could have avoided the aspiration pneumonia. I felt guilty for her suffering.

But there was no looking back now. At least I knew my instincts were right. All I could hope for was that a Chiari decompression surgery would solve her difficulties.

It's hard when you have twins and one with special needs not to compare them. Sophia was already walking, eating solids, and babbling. She was an overall happy child, very independent and with a bubbly personality.

Alessia, on the other hand, was always sick. She couldn't help it. For her it was a huge milestone to be able to swallow a few drops of water without aspirating. To be able to coordinate her legs and arms to crawl took so much strength and practice. They were on two opposite ends of the developmental spectrum, and it was heartbreaking to watch. What Sophia did with no effort at all would cost so much for Alessia. Slowly but surely, I thought. If I could just get Alessia's Chiari decompressed she would catch up to her sister. I knew she would.

The appointment with neurosurgery was scheduled for July 29, 2016.

We tried to enjoy our summer. I got the girls a kiddie pool for them to play in and they loved it. We went out on my stepdad's boat on Lake Norman often. Thiago was getting to be a pro at diving off the boat into the water. Sophia enjoyed floating in the water in her floatie and Alessia loved having water poured on her head while she sat in her walker. Every outing on the boat was therapeutic.

I felt a sense of normalcy when I went on that boat—it gave me a break from having to brainstorm ways to keep my daughter alive. It's those small breaks that give you the energy to continue. The time you can just sit back and enjoy the moment where everyone is actually "living," because you can get so tied up on trying to make life "normal" when "normal" for a family raising a medically complex child is so very abnormal.

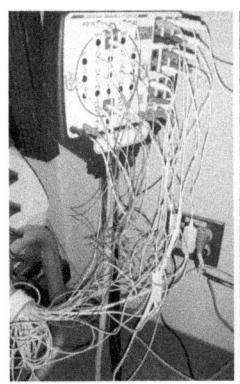
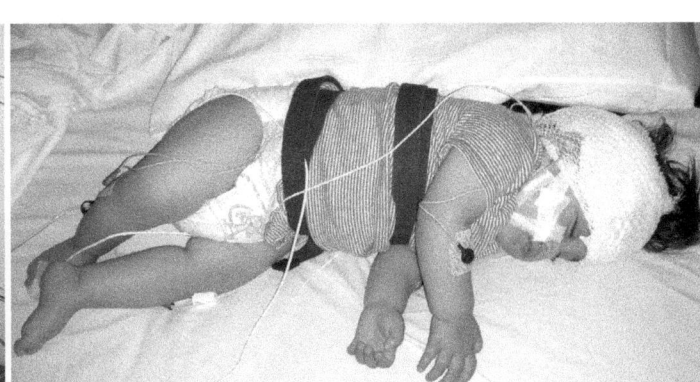

*Sleep study cables*          *Alessia's sleep study, 2016*
*Both Photo Credits: Stephanie Detjen Costabel*

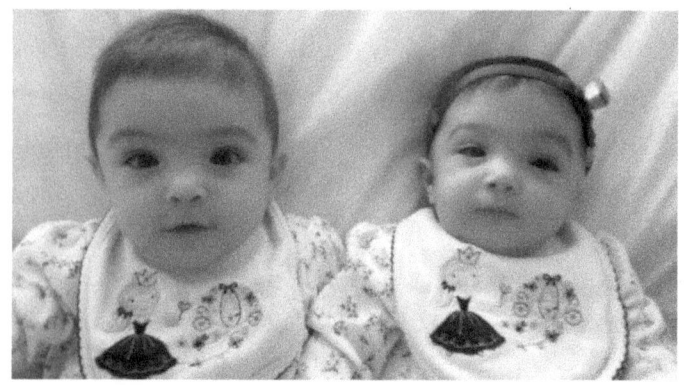

*Sophia and Alessia, 2015*

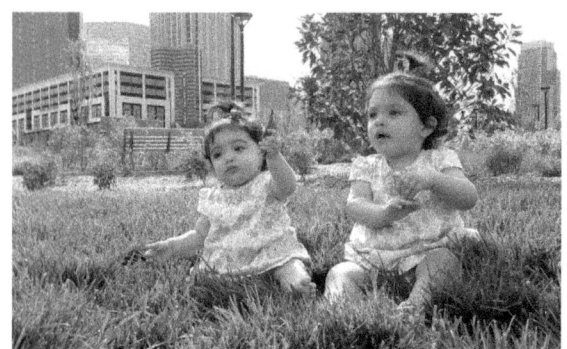

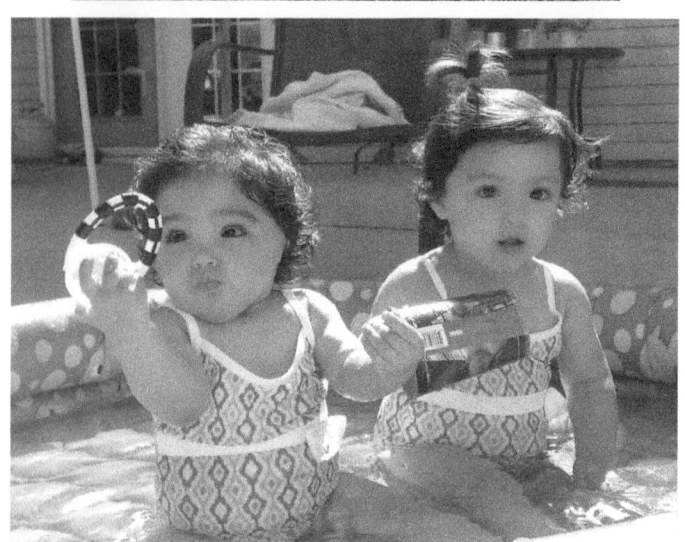

*Alessia and Sophia, Summer 2016*
*All Photos Credits: Stephanie Detjen Costabel*

## 12

I researched as much as I possibly could about Chiari malformation. I spent my nights reading medical articles on my phone about the condition while my family slept. I came across a Chiari Facebook group that I joined to get advice from other Chiarians.

I researched the pros and cons of decompression surgery. I even saw a video of an actual decompression surgery on YouTube. It probably was not the best thing I could have done, because the procedure looked painful and invasive. It's amazing how the internet can fill you with information. The more I read about Chiari and decompression surgery, the more convinced I was that Alessia would benefit from this surgery.

I had been warned by other Chiari mothers that it would be a battle to get a good Chiari expert neurosurgeon and to have them intervene surgically. I had daily contact with Deanna from the RES Facebook page who put me in contact with her son's neurosurgeon out in California: Dr. Gerald Grant. He was the best of the best according to Deanna and the Chiari group. I wanted to get his opinion before I met with our local neurosurgeon. It was going to be difficult for us to travel to California for an in-person appointment, though, so I called his office and explained the situation to them. They gave me his email address after he agreed to look at Alessia's case.

I sent him an email with a recap of where we were medically.

My fingers trembled as I clicked "Send."

The politics in healthcare suggests the most professional way to be seen is to schedule an appointment with a provider and discuss health issues face-to-face. But I didn't have time for that: I was ten days out from my local neurosurgeon's appointment and there was just no way I could jump on a plane with Alessia to see Dr. Grant before then. If my local neurosurgery appointment didn't go well and if they did not offer decompression surgery, then my next step would be to travel to California to see Dr. Grant.

I was incredibly surprised when the following day I got a call from his office to notify me he would look at Alessia's scans. That same day, I overnighted Alessia's MRI CDs.

Now it was just a waiting game. I really hoped he would answer before our appointment with our local neurosurgeon.

I wanted my mother and Ronaldo to come with me. I wanted all of us there to hear what the neurosurgeon was going to say. I printed out her sleep study results, ABR hearing test, swallowing study results, and took videos of Alessia dragging her head on the floor, which was common head pain behavior for a child with Chiari. I practiced in front of the mirror what I was going to tell our neurosurgeon if he decided not to do the decompression surgery. The night before our appointment I could not sleep. When you have a child with such rare brain malformations, and doctors that can't even pronounce Rhombencephalosynapsis, you worry about the fight ahead.

I got up early and got dressed like I was going to a job interview. I wanted to look professional and educated, so the neurosurgeon would take my concerns seriously. My mother dressed her best as well as Ronaldo. I put matching outfits on the twins. They were adorable.

My mother tried to calm me down by assuring me he had not said "no" to the decompression surgery yet. I needed to relax, but I could not. It was ninety degrees outside, but my hands were cold, and I couldn't stop cracking my knuckles. My hands get cold and fidgety when I am nervous.

We walked into Carolina Neurosurgery & Spine Associates. We were impressed by how nice the clinic was. I admired the modern abstract paintings hanging on the walls. The waiting area and lobby faced huge windows overlooking the outdoors with plants and flowers and greenery. There was a beautiful saltwater fish tank in the waiting area as well as modern sofas with plenty of magazines and books on the side tables. There was also a children's waiting area that had children-sized chairs and tables. I was impressed by the modern look of the clinic.

We sat down in the lobby while I filled out the forms. Not even ten minutes went by when I heard, "Alessia Cruz." They were ready for us. The physician assistant looked young. Once in a room, she sat in front of the computer in the room and started asking us all kinds of questions. Symptoms, medications, medical history, etc. We spent about thirty minutes going over all Alessia's medical issues. She then measured Alessia's head circumference. "Dr. Van Poppel will be in here shortly," she said, and exited the room.

Dr. Van Poppel walked into the room after what seemed like fifteen minutes. He looked young for a neurosurgeon, probably in his mid-thirties. He greeted us and shook each our hands.

He went straight to the point. He showed us Alessia's MRI scans on the computer and explained to us how her Chiari was rather tight and recommended a decompression surgery.

My jaw dropped to the floor. I didn't have to fight! I didn't have to explain absolutely anything! Dr. Van Poppel was on the same page as we were. His recommendations were decompression surgery because her Chiari was rather significant, which was totally different from what her neurologist had told me over the phone a few weeks ago.

He wanted to do the decompression surgery sooner rather than later. He explained his goal was for her sleep apnea and swallowing difficulties to improve after decompression. He would only do a bony decompression, which would involve shaving some bone from the bottom of her skull to give the cerebellum more space. He would not open the dura. Post-surgery was going to be a four-to-five-day hospital stay. I had spent so much time worrying about this appointment and how it would go badly and how I would have to argue to get him to decompress. He suddenly became my best friend.

My mother, Ronaldo, and I looked at each other with wide eyes. We were all speechless. "Any questions?" Dr. Van Poppel asked.

I was speechless, so happy and relieved. "Uh, no," I gulped. We left that appointment and as soon as we got into the car, I realized that I needed to chill.

"You did all that worrying . . . all that research, you had nightmares about this appointment, practiced speeches in the mirror . . . FOR NO REASON! You really need to take a chill pill and relax," Ronaldo said, chuckling.

I agreed, but also knew without my persistence we wouldn't be where we were. I glanced at my Alessia, and she was just staring at me smiling.

That same day, Dr. Van Poppel's physician assistant called me to schedule the decompression surgery. The date was set, August 4, 2016. Next week! I had six days to plan everything. The childcare of Sophia and Thiago, my hospital stay for four days with Alessia, and making sure everything at home was ready for my absence . . . laundry, housework, groceries, cleaning, etc.

Ronaldo had to work but was going to work half days. Between my mother, him, and my sisters (Jatrin and Kassandra), we were all going to help and make it work. I was going to do the night shifts. Ronaldo, my mother, and my sisters were going to take turns during the day to stay with Alessia at the hospital.

The weekend before the surgery we decided to enjoy the beautiful summer weather. My mother and I took the girls and Thiago to Romare Bearden Park on a beautiful Sunday afternoon. In the late afternoons the shade from the downtown buildings provided a relief from the sun. The warm summer breeze hugged my body.

Romare Bearden Park is a plaza with beautiful green grass out in the open, surrounded by the towers of uptown Charlotte. It has water fountains that light up red, blue, and yellow when the sun sets. All colors were intertwined and steadily faded away . . . turquoise, purple, and shades of orange ending in the beginning of the darkness of the night. It was a breathtaking view.

Ronaldo had gifted me a professional camera for my birthday. I had never used it before that day at the park. I was going to capture the moments of our girls and son enjoying the beautiful day. I dressed the girls in matching white summer dresses. I put white jasmine flower clips on their short, curly, baby hair. Thiago had on a pair of khaki slacks with a white, coastal beach shirt. He looked so handsome for a five-year-old boy. He was going to be a heartbreaker for sure when he is older, I thought. They smiled, laughed, and enjoyed the wonderful summer evening. Thiago skipped and did flips on the grass. The warm summer sunset helped make the photographs I took a masterpiece of art. All three of them were in great spirits and had a joyful mood. I enjoyed watching their young innocent spirits—we should all learn from the simple ways children entertain themselves.

Secretly I was preparing myself for Alessia's decompression surgery. But I kept reminding myself you must stop and smell the flowers. You must learn to enjoy the present moment, especially when your medically complex child is happy. It was hard to do knowing that my daughter was going to go into brain surgery in a matter of hours. But smelling the flowers and enjoying the present moment is the fuel that helps keep you going. These are the moments you hold on to and remember. You cannot change your situation, but you can learn to live with your situation. The grass felt fresh underneath the soles of my feet. Alessia couldn't walk yet but was crawling around looking and picking at the rich green colored grass. Each photo I took, each minute of happiness I witnessed of my children laughing and enjoying themselves in that park, will forever hold a place in my heart.

August 4: I woke up, put some comfortable clothes on, and carried Alessia into her car seat while she was still asleep. We had to be at Levine Children's Hospital at 6 a.m. She was the first case. Jatrin met Alessia and me at the hospital. My mother stayed taking care of Sophia and Thiago while Ronaldo went to work. Kassandra was going to come the following day to help stay with Alessia at the hospital.

When I arrived, there was a line at the front desk, as all surgeries went through the same check-in process. I observed the other children in line. Most of the babies were accompanied by nervous parents. We did not know each other but we shared the same anguish. One little boy caught my eye—he was about four years old and in a wheelchair wearing Spiderman pajamas. His breathing sounded labored and wet. I watched as his mother carefully pulled out a suction machine and connected it to his tracheostomy. With the press of a button, she turned on the machine and suctioned out his secretions. Within a matter of seconds his breathing returned to normal again. I wondered how often she had to press that suction machine. I stopped to think how many times a day we swallow our own saliva. To a person who did not have the capability of swallowing, that meant that every time he needed to swallow, he would need to be suctioned out by a machine. I quickly looked away and wiped a tear off with my finger.

That could be Alessia, I thought. That could have been me suctioning out her secretions.

It is incredible how much we take for granted. To be able to swallow is a blessing. To not be connected to machines to live on this Earth is a gift. Some people don't have that gift. The taste of salty crackers with cheese, ice cream with chocolate syrup, the refreshment you feel in your throat when you take a gulp of icy water, a lick of the sweetness of a lollipop, the luxury of taste, all things children with dysphagia could not experience.

I just hoped this surgery would help Alessia. The hope for improvement in her condition. I needed faith. My faith in God had been deteriorating.

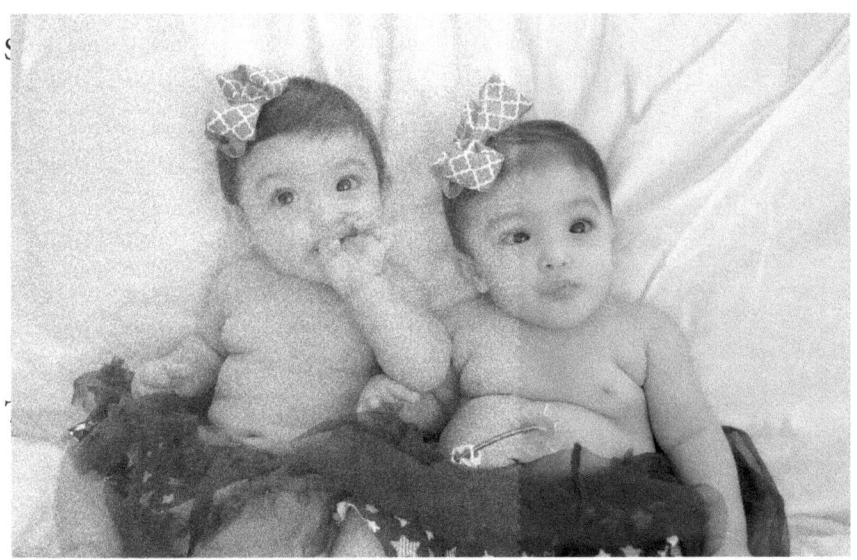

*Sophia and Alessia. Alessia still had her PEG tube in this photo.*
*Photo Credit: Stephanie Detjen Costabel*

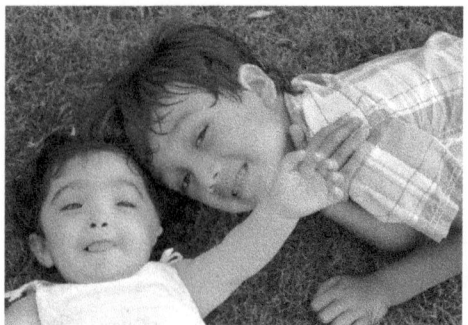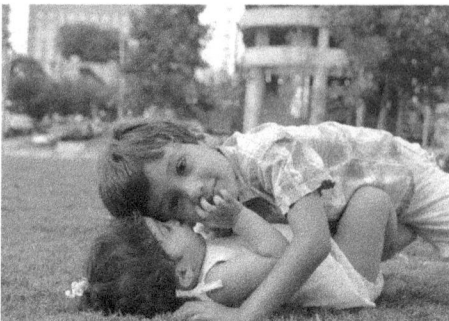

*Thiago and Alessia at Romare Bearden Park, 2016*

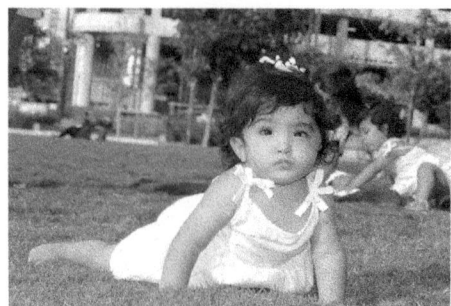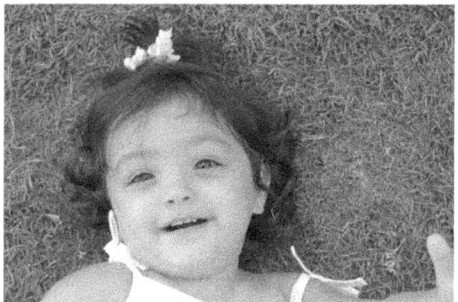

*Sophia at Romare Bearden Park, 2016*

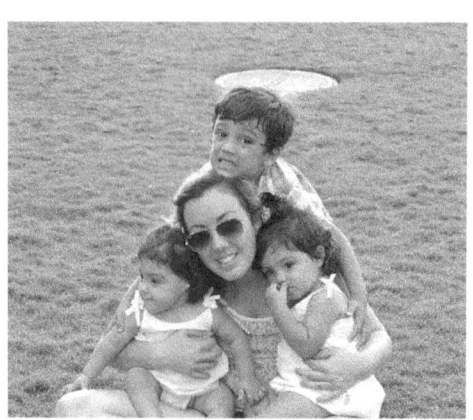

*Thiago, Sophia, Alessia, and me.*
*Romare Bearden Park, 2016*
*All pics Photo Credit:*
*Stephanie Detjen Costabel*

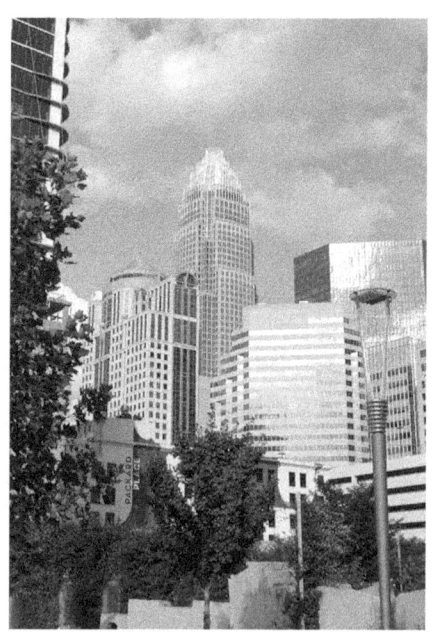

## 13

Four hours later the decompression surgery had been completed. Dr. Van Poppel walked into the conference room to talk to my sister and me. The same conference room we had been to many times already. The room is supposed to be comforting in case you were thrown bad news from the surgeons.

"Everything went well," Dr. Van Poppel said with enthusiasm. "We were able to do a good bony decompression. We had no problems at all. She did very well. The only thing is that anesthesia had a difficult time intubating her. The anatomy of her airway is abnormal, so they decided to keep her intubated tonight to make sure everything goes well with her recovery. We will give her some time to rest and if everything goes well tonight, she should be able to be extubated tomorrow morning. She'll be in pediatric ICU today until she is extubated."

I could feel my palms start to sweat. Still intubated?? PICU?? I could feel my stomach getting queasy.

Dr. Van Poppel probably could tell I was petrified. "This is only for precaution," he assured me. "She did very well, but there's also risks of complication right after surgery. We just want to make sure she goes through the next twenty-four hours without any events and if everything goes well, she will be extubated in the morning. Hang in there, Mom."

He smiled and walked out of the conference room.

I had seen my daughter intubated lying on a hospital bed many times before. I should have already been used to the view. But it still hurt. No matter how many times you see your child lying in a hospital bed, the feeling of helplessness and sadness does not get easier.

The rest of the afternoon, I just sat next to her hospital bed and held her hand. She was completely sedated. I prayed hard. Although by that point my faith in prayer had already begun to decline.

She had an uneventful night. Everything pointed towards a successful extubation in the morning. Extubation is often difficult to watch since they must wean off her sedation. As she started to wake up the breathing tube was uncomfortable, and she would try to yank it out. The respiratory therapist, ICU doctor, and anesthesia all had to be in the room for extubation, especially with her since she had an abnormal airway. If thirty minutes went by and not everyone was ready, they would have to sedate her again for a couple of minutes. At around 11 a.m., everybody was ready to extubate. I usually wait outside of the room since it's too nerve-wracking to watch. I felt like I was going to throw up.

"Extubation successful, Mom!" the nurse smiled as she walked out of the room.

I let out a sigh of relief, as my heart and breathing returned to normal. "Thank you, God," I whispered to myself. When I went in, Alessia was in good spirits. I quickly picked her up and got a glimpse at her incision. It looked so painful. It extended from the lower portion of her head all the way down her neck. It looked like at least twenty stitches, but I didn't want to count. I looked at Alessia's face and couldn't help to think how incredible she was. She was smiling and babbling as though nothing had happened. I wondered if her head pain from her Chiari had been so severe that now she felt relief after being decompressed. Either way, I was extremely impressed and relieved by how well she handled the surgery.

Four days later, we were ready to go home. Alessia's recovery at the hospital was miraculous. She was such an inspiration. I was so proud of her. Everything looked up for us. Her incision was healing nicely. Everything was going as planned. Everything will start to improve, I thought.

The night she was discharged from the hospital after her decompression surgery was the first night in months that I slept like a baby. I was happy and relieved and loved the feeling of sleeping in my own bed.

The following few weeks went by uneventfully. Alessia was in good spirits. She even started crawling. Her muscle coordination was better than ever. She was sleeping well through the night, and I even noticed that her pulse oximeter machine wasn't alarming as much as before surgery.

We had regular eye appointments to check her optic nerves and corneal health. Dr. Daugherty was her local ophthalmologist in Charlotte. He was a charming man with excellent bedside manners, showing concern for Alessia's well-being. He had seen her since birth, checking Sophia and Alessia for retina of prematurity. He had referred us to Duke Eye Center when Alessia's corneal ulcer wasn't healing, but for regular checkup appointments we always went to him. "Hi, everybody," he cheerfully said as he walked into the examination room. He was so good with kids. "Wow, she looks great! I'm so glad she is doing this good. She certainly is a fighter."

I smiled.

"Now let's just make sure those optic nerves are looking flat."

I had dilated her eyes at home, so I anticipated the visit was going to be a quick one. I wasn't nervous or anxious or anything. And since she was doing so good, I doubted there was anything wrong with her optic nerves. I had put a wine bottle in the freezer before I left. I was looking forward to a romantic evening with Ronaldo. I held Alessia on my lap while Dr. Daugherty opened each eye with a speculum. She never liked the eye exams and would always fuss when they propped her eye open, which gave me the impression her eyeball would pop out. Dr. Daugherty always assured me she would not feel any pain since she did not have sensation in the corneas. The room was silent while Alessia cried for a little bit and between his assistant and me we held her down. Dr. Daugherty took longer than usual observing her optic nerves. That was uncommon. My heart started racing as I tried not to ask him what was wrong. He furrowed his eyebrows and bit his lower lip. Suddenly he appeared worried.

"What's wrong?" my voice trembled. "What did you see?"

"Well . . ." Long pause. "Her optic nerves are swollen. More so than the last time I saw them." He took the speculum out of Alessia's eyes and put it away. "I'm sorry to say this, but I do believe her intracranial pressure might be elevated. I think it would be a good idea for you to take her to the ER."

Fuck! I thought. "Wait. What? How is that even possible? We just decompressed her Chiari less than two months ago?"

"Yes, I understand. But you can have permanent vision loss with her optic nerves being as swollen as they are for an extended period of time. I recommend you head to the hospital."

I couldn't believe this was happening. I glanced at Alessia, and she was looking at me with an innocent look in her eyes. She could not understand what was going on. She did not look sick.

"I will call Dr. Van Poppel and let him know. Keep me updated on what they say," Dr. Daugherty said as he exited the room.

*This can't be happening. It was supposed to be a routine eye exam, not a trip to the ER . . .*

I had both girls with me. I called Ronaldo in tears. "Baby, Dr. Daugherty has just sent us to the ER. Alessia's optic nerves are swollen. Could you please come get Sophia at Levine?" I gulped as I tried to stay calm.

"What?!?" he asked.

I hated the ER. You never know what to expect there. I've learned throughout the years that in the ER you can have a life-threatening situation in a matter of minutes or nothing wrong at all. Those are some of the obstacles you face when you have a non-verbal child. They can't tell you what hurts so it's a guessing game. The ER runs tests trying to rule out potential medical causes for pain, and when they find nothing, you get sent home with a fussy child that can't tell you what's wrong.

I walked into the children's emergency room petrified. I checked in and they quickly led me to the back where the rooms were. I had both girls with me in their car seats. Ronaldo called and was about ten minutes away. The ER had been alerted that I was coming. I felt heat running through my veins as I tried to hold back my tears. I was so angry, sad, nervous, and anxious, all at the same time. Life was so unfair for Alessia! She had just recovered from decompression surgery and here she was less than two months later with God knows what other issue.

After about an hour of waiting, Dr. Van Poppel's PA came to our ER room. "Hey there!" The look in her eyes told me she was worried.

"What's going on?" I asked. "I went to a simple routine eye exam. The eye doctor told me Alessia's optic nerves were swollen and sent me here. Can you explain to me what the concern is?"

"Yes. Dr. Daugherty called our office, concerned about your daughter's optic nerves. She showed severe papilledema in the exam today. The plan is to get a sedated Chiari protocol MRI and CINE flow study again," she said. She measured Alessia' s head and felt her decompression surgery area. "Didn't we just do this three months ago?" I asked. I was fuming.

"We did, yes, but we only did a bony decompression surgery. We thought that would be enough. We did not open the dura. We try to avoid opening the dura, but sometimes it's necessary. If the MRI shows she's still tight there, we will have to have another decompression surgery with a duraplasty. Basically, this translates to opening up the dura and patching a graft to make more space for the cerebellum."

"Why didn't we do this the first time around?" I tried to keep Alessia calm—she was tired of being there, I could tell.

"Well, we try to avoid opening the dura unless we absolutely have to. Dr. Van Poppel would like to have this MRI done on Monday when all of anesthesia's staff will be here . . . just as a precaution since she's got a difficult airway. So, the plan is to admit her for the weekend so we can monitor her, and Monday morning we will go into that Chiari MRI and do the duraplasty surgery if necessary."

"What?!?" I asked. My voice was higher pitched than normal. I couldn't hold back my anger. "Why would we have to stay for two days? She's perfectly fine. She and I both are going to go crazy in this hospital until Monday!" My heart was racing at that point, and I could feel I was losing my cool.

"I know it's an inconvenience for you to be here over the weekend . . ."

"NO!" I interrupted her. "It's not an inconvenience for me. It's the fact of her staying here for two days when you guys aren't even going to do anything until Monday. I mean look at her! She's perfectly fine. She's laughing, but obviously sick of being here and she's moving around. What could possibly go wrong?" I was fighting back the tears. I already had PTSD from being in the hospital.

"I understand." She got up from her seat. "Let me talk to Dr. Van Poppel. For now, let's get you up to a room and see if we can do anything that would be easier on you guys for the next two days."

I couldn't contain my frustration and anguish and started crying.

"Please! I just don't want to stay here with her at this hospital. Let her enjoy her weekend at home and we will come back on Monday and get everything done." I buried my face in my hands.

"Let's see what we can do," she said as she exited the ER room.

After about two hours there was finally a room upstairs for us. By then it was already 8 p.m. I had to wait until I had an update from neurosurgery. Alessia was extremely irritable. She was rubbing her eyes and acting extremely fussy. I could tell she did not want to be there.

I was sweating trying to keep her entertained while she was ripping out her leads they had put on her in the ER. Alessia was a fighter. She was strong. She definitely let us know what she wanted and what she did not. That night she did not want to be there.

About an hour later, Dr. Van Poppel entered the room. He looked extremely tired. I could tell his day had been busy. "Hey, Mom, I know you don't want to be here, so I've thought of what can make it easier for you. I can't do the MRI and surgery this weekend because I want to have everyone from anesthesia at the hospital on Monday morning since she is such a difficult intubation. During the weekend, we don't have as much staff compared to a weekday. So, I went ahead and scheduled a sedated Chiari protocol MRI with CINE flow study for Monday morning, and afterwards we will keep her intubated. If she needs to have another decompression surgery with a duraplasty, which I strongly think she will need, then we will go ahead and do it Monday morning after the MRI." He glanced at Alessia and saw how she was yanking at her leads. "Now I know it's going to be difficult to keep her calm this weekend here at the hospital, so to make it easier on you guys, I will prescribe Diamox throughout the weekend to lower her ICP [intracranial pressure] and that way you can go home tonight and just come back Monday morning . . . Sound like a plan?" he asked.

I let out a sigh of relief. I wish he would have done the duraplasty from the get-go, but at the same time I completely understood why he only did a bony decompression first. I could tell he was trying to keep us as comfortable as possible, and I appreciated that. "Thank you so much, Dr. Van Poppel, I truly appreciate it," I said as I comforted my crying Alessia.

We were home by midnight. Ronaldo had put Sophia and Thiago to sleep and was anxiously waiting for us by the front door. "So, explain to me with more detail what happened today, you didn't make sense on the phone."

"I'm so sorry," I said as I hugged him. "I have been so nervous and a total emotional wreck all day. I don't even recall what I said on the phone. Alessia has swollen optic nerves. They call it papilledema. The buildup of cerebral spinal fluid in the brain causes her optic nerves to swell. She most likely will require more decompression on her Chiari, but Dr. Van Poppel let us go home tonight. We need to go again on Monday morning to do the Chiari protocol MRI and then the surgery, which he thinks is what needs to be done." A tear ran down my cheek. The incision that was so nicely healed up would have to be reopened. This time more invasive surgery to decompress. Ronaldo just looked down and covered his face with his hands. We both quietly went upstairs to our room and tried to go to sleep.

Jatrin was getting married the following week. If Alessia's decompression surgery was like last time, we would most likely have to stay four days at the hospital, making her discharge day right on my sister's wedding. I was the maid of honor, and Sophia and Alessia were the flower girls. My family from Uruguay was coming for the wedding. I had looked forward to dressing the twins in beautiful white flower girl dresses. I was not going to ask my sister to cancel her wedding since she had been planning it for a whole year. But I was sad that Alessia and I were not going to be able to make it.

## An Amazing Little Girl with Rhombencephalosynapsis

I took a quick shower, cleaned up Alessia, who was drifting off to sleep by then, and lay on my bed. I closed my tired eyes but could not sleep. I tossed and turned, my heart racing, my body shivering. I could not control my anxiety and restlessness. Finally, at 2 a.m., I went downstairs and poured myself a glass of the wine I had previously put in the refrigerator. So much for the romantic night I had planned with Ronaldo.

I smoked cigarettes every so often but hadn't in a long time. I sat on the front porch with my glass of wine and lit up a cigarette that I had saved from months before. I didn't want to get into the habit of drinking and smoking, but that night I needed it. I seriously questioned God's existence. Everybody would tell me: God only gives you what you can handle. Bullshit, if that were the case than there wouldn't be suicide, I thought. They would tell me God chooses special mothers to be caregivers of special-needs children. They would say I was strong and that they would not know what to do in my situation. I even had some people tell me Alessia came to this world to teach us a lesson. A lesson? What the hell? People were ridiculous. The truth was I was not strong, I was a concerned and loving mother. I was surviving the situation that I was in. I did not believe that God gave me this situation for some mysterious reason that I had to learn from or find my purpose. I started to understand that "shit happens." There was no religious reason behind it. I could not imagine God sitting on his throne in heaven just handing me down these difficult situations and allowing my daughter to go through all the suffering in order to prove a point or make me learn a lesson.

So, I sat there drinking my wine and smoking my cigarette, as my whole concept of God started to shift.

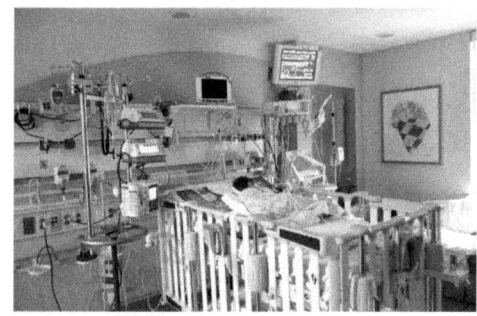

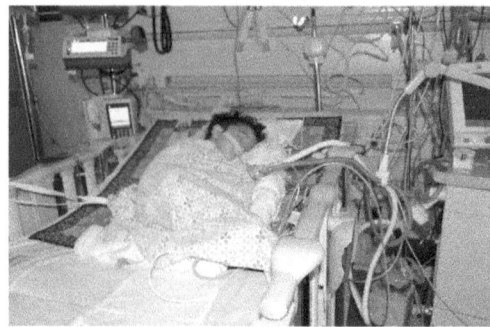

*Alessia's PICU room at Levine after her decompression surgery, August 2016*

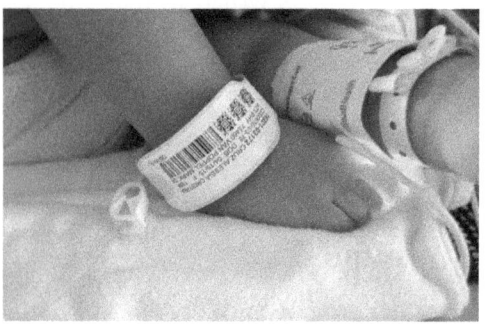

*Alessia at the PICU after her decompression surgery, August 2016
All pics Photo Credit: Stephanie Detjen Costabel*

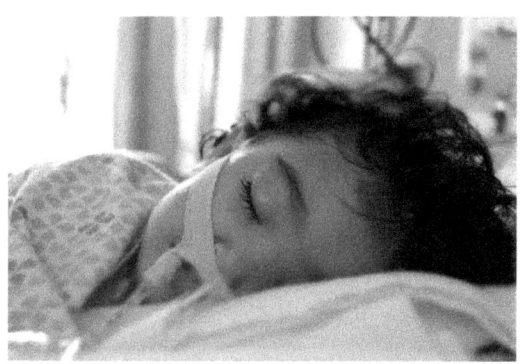

## 14

Monday morning came faster than I wanted. We had to be at Levine at 6 a.m. Alessia was the first scheduled for an MRI.

October mornings were starting to become chilly. Ronaldo heated up the van before I got Alessia up and into her car seat. He kissed me goodbye and then kissed Alessia's cheek. "I love you." I could hear him whispering in her ear. He turned towards me. "Good luck, baby, call me as soon she goes back." A tear ran down my cheek. Part of me wished he would go with me, but someone had to stay with Thiago and Sophia. Children were not allowed in the PICU. Thiago was going to go to school so he would be entertained, but Sophia was staying with Ronaldo until my mother got off work. She would stay with Sophia and wait for Thiago to come home from school, so Ronaldo could go to the hospital.

The sun was starting to rise as I drove down Independence Boulevard. Orange, red, and yellow colors filled the horizon. The uptown high-rises reflected the sun's early rays.

I had spent the weekend pretending everything was fine for the sake of my children and my family. Everybody was excited for my sister's wedding. We had not seen our family from Uruguay for over two years. My sister was trying so hard to focus on her wedding, but she was also concerned about Alessia's surgery. I tried to reassure everybody that everything was going to be okay and to not worry.

The pretending game.

Only mothers of special-needs children understand that game. You pretend everything is fine, when deep down inside you are hurting, heartbroken, and worried. You do it because you want to maintain normalcy for the people you love. Especially to your other children, who by no fault of their own must deal with the side effects of the situation, like your constant exhaustion, bad mood, and lack of energy. The pretending game becomes a daily thing, so nobody you love hurts the way you do. Special-needs mothers are great at the pretending game.

We were led to the third floor—Radiology. After pre-op came and talked to me and all forms were signed, I was led back to the MRI room. Anesthesia was waiting for me there since surgery was not going to be done until Dr. Van Poppel reviewed the scans. I was able to be with her until anesthesia sedated her. After the MRI, she would stay intubated until Dr. Van Poppel reviewed the scans and went from there.

I kissed her soft cheek goodbye and whispered "I love you" in her tiny microtia ear as anesthesia put the gas mask on and she drifted to sleep. Then I was led to the waiting room. I knew the drill. I had been there many times before. The receptionists all knew me there, which was nice. It didn't feel so lonely. Two hours later, I was led to the same conference room as always to talk to Dr. Van Poppel.

"Hey there," he smiled as he walked in the room. "MRI is done. I reviewed her scans, and her Chiari is still quite tight. As I had suspected, she needs to have another decompression surgery with a duraplasty. It's a little more invasive since we have to open the dura and sew on a graft to make more room for the cerebellum. But it's the same process as last time... a four-night hospital stay... probably keeping her intubated overnight in the PICU and extubate her in the morning if everything goes well."

I nodded as a tear ran down my cheek.

"I'll come get you once the procedure is done, okay? Anticipate approximately four hours. Hang in there, Mom."

My sister Kassandra brought me lunch and stayed with me for a few hours. Then came Ronaldo. We would take frequent breaks from that waiting room and go outside to get some fresh air. It's incredible how being at the hospital consumes you. The hours feel endless while you sit and wait. I had been in that waiting room since 8 a.m. I noticed there were some parents that had gotten there earlier than me and were still waiting. Some slept, some read books, some scrolled down their phones. We were all sharing the same anguish.

Finally, around 4 p.m. the receptionist called Alessia's name and led us to the familiar conference room. Ronaldo and I tried to stay calm while we waited for Dr. Van Poppel to come talk to us. My hands were cold. My stomach felt queasy.

*What is wrong with me? I should be used to this by now.*

"What's wrong, baby? You look pale. Just relax, everything is going to be okay," Ronaldo said as he held my hand.

"Hey there," I heard. Dr. Van Poppel walked in. "She did well! We did a pretty big decompression and duraplasty. I had to shave off some excess bone that had grown back from the last decompression. She's doing well! Hang in there."

*God, he always says the same thing when he leaves.* I chuckled.

We were taken to the PICU. Alessia lay in the same position as after last surgery and coincidentally was in the same PICU room. The PICU team remembered her. She was hard to forget given her complex medical history. Her beauty attracted anyone who saw her. Her eyelashes were long and dark. She had an abundance of dark thick hair. "Look at all that hair," the nurses would say. She had the cutest, tiniest button nose and chubby cheeks. Alessia was beautiful indeed. A tear ran down my cheek, grateful she was okay.

The following morning, she was extubated successfully and transferred to Progressive Care. As always, she was doing amazingly well with her recovery . . . so much so that they let us go home a day early.

I did not have much help during that hospital stay, because my mother was busy with my family from Uruguay, and my sisters were busy with last-minute arrangements for Jatrin's wedding. So, I was exhausted when we were discharged. We got home around 4 p.m. The wedding was the following day, and I had to be at the venue at 11 a.m. I needed to make sure my dress and shoes were ready, and I had absolutely no idea what I was going to do with my crazy hair. It was too late to make an appointment at the salon for the next morning.

I walked over to the girls' closet. I went to the back where their flower-girl dresses hung gracefully. I took out Sophia's dress and hung it on the doorknob. I took out Alessia's dress and could feel the urge to cry running through my veins. I couldn't hold it back and fell to my knees. "Oh God, I can't take her!" I sobbed uncontrollably. There was just no way. Her incision was a little larger than last time and she had only just left the hospital. I couldn't take her and expose her to all those people. She was still fragile. I sobbed thinking she would not get to wear her beautiful flower-girl dress and be a part of the wedding. I wanted to be there for my sister, but at the same time I needed to be there for my daughter.

I felt Ronaldo's hand wrap around me. He knew what I was feeling. "I know how important this is for you," he said as he kissed my cheek. "You have to go to your sister's wedding. I asked my sister to come take care of Alessia tomorrow so we can go to the wedding."

"But I don't want to leave her!" I cried. The guilt I felt was drowning me. I could do nothing but sob, clinging onto my husband's shoulder. There weren't any words that would make me feel better. Just having a shoulder to cry on until I could cry no more was somewhat relieving.

I was beyond tired, but Alessia was uncomfortable from the surgery. She had narcotics prescribed for pain as well as muscle relaxers. Every three to four hours I would administer her meds through her tube, as well as check her incision for any drainage or signs of infection. Even with all her medications, she was still restless. How could she not be when she'd just had brain surgery for the second time in two months?

I got up at 8 a.m. the following day. I had two hours to get ready and leave everything ready for my sister-in-law so she could attend to Alessia's medical needs. I felt terrible. I couldn't believe I was leaving my daughter to go to my sister's wedding. I owed it to my sister, though she would have been okay if I had decided not to go.

Thiago looked as cute as can be with his khaki slacks and white button-down shirt. He had a cute coral-colored bow tie, and his shiny brown shoes made him look so grown up. When did my boy get so big? Sophia looked like a princess with her white puffy flower-girl dress that extended to her calves. She had white tights and the cutest ballerina shoes. I secured a white flower hair clip to the side of her baby hair. She was the prettiest flower girl I had ever laid eyes on.

Ronaldo looked handsome in his khaki slacks and matching vest and also had a coral-colored bow tie. It was nice to see him so dressed up—it had been more than a year since we had dressed up so nicely. I, on the other hand, looked and felt terrible. The bags under my eyes extended down to my cheeks. I looked like I hadn't slept in ages. No matter how much concealer I put on, I couldn't hide the exhaustion. My skin felt rough and tired. My wrinkles were visible.

By the time I finished getting Thiago and Sophia ready and prepared all of Alessia's feeds and meds for my sister-in-law, I had fifteen minutes to do something to my frizzy hair. I pulled it back in a messy bun and tried to secure stray strands with bobby pins. It looked like I had just left the gym. I tried not to focus on how bad I looked. I was more concerned about how Alessia would do with my sister-in-law. I had written a schedule on what times she needed to be fed and what times to administer her meds. My sister-in-law had only fed her a few times through her tube, but she seemed comfortable with it. Or at least she showed me she was. *It will only be a few hours. Alessia probably won't even notice that I'm gone. She will be in good hands. My sister-in-law will take good care of her . . .* I tried to hold back my tears.

It was a beautiful October day—a perfect day to get married. Thankfully, it was not cold, and there wasn't a cloud in the sky. I had missed the preparation with all of the bridesmaids and also the photos of my sister and her bridesmaids getting their hair and makeup done. I wish I could have been there with my sister to have shared that experience with her. All the bridesmaids looked beautiful and here I was, the maid of honor, looking like I had just left the gym.

I couldn't complain, though; at least Alessia wasn't discharged on my sister's wedding day and thank God she had no complications. At the end of the day, that is what I was thankful for. It just killed me she couldn't be there with us.

I called my sister-in-law to check up on Alessia at least ten times throughout the wedding. "She is perfectly fine," she assured me every time I called. Even with the reassurance I still felt nervous. It wasn't that I didn't believe my sister-in-law, but it was the permanent guilt I felt of Alessia not being at the wedding.

My sister looked stunning. Her youth glowed from afar. She was so beautiful and so happy. She was so appreciative that I had come to the wedding, albeit feeling sad for her niece, but she hid it well. At the end of the day, I was glad she hadn't canceled the wedding. Everyone seemed to be enjoying themselves and Thiago and Sophia were having fun running around the venue.

The reception went quickly, which was good for me since I was anxious to get back home to Alessia. My family from Uruguay decided to come over to my house after the reception so they could see Alessia and spend time with her.

"She did well, she just wanted to be held constantly," my sister-in-law said as she got up from the couch and started heading out. I scooped Alessia up in my arms and planted a large kiss on her forehead. "I missed you," I whispered in her microtia ear. I got the impression she understood what was going on. As soon as she saw we were all back home, she didn't want to be carried anymore. "I'm so sorry, mami, please forgive me," I said out loud and stroked her hair.

"They're here!" Ronaldo said as he walked into the dining room. My grandmother and uncles from Uruguay walked through the front door with bags of groceries. Oh Lord, I thought. They are probably going to do a cookout.

I was happy to see my family since I hadn't seen them for so long, but I was just so exhausted and tired that all I really wanted was to sleep. I handed Alessia over to my mother and went to the bathroom to wash my face. As I looked at myself in the mirror, I tried to fake a smile. Time to pretend, I said to myself.

Throughout the years I have learned how to fake a smile to bring normalcy to my family while I am dying inside. I could have been a Hollywood actress. To the world I was happy. I cracked jokes for my children to be happy . . . I had romantic nights with my husband to have some normalcy in our marriage. I tried to take care of my physical appearance so I wouldn't look unkempt. In reality, I cared two shits about how I looked.

Time to pretend. Again.

You pretend to enjoy life while you feel guilty because your child cannot. The helplessness that you cannot change what you cannot control. The endless guilt. Everything made me feel guilty. How could I enjoy the taste of my favorite meal when I knew Alessia could not taste food? How could I enjoy the sound of my favorite music when I knew Alessia could not hear? How could I enjoy a pain-free life when I knew my daughter was always sick and in pain? You become an expert at pretending . . . to pretend that life was magical and beautiful and joyful. It took years for me to learn that you can be happy, that life is indeed beautiful, and that special-needs parenting can be magical and rewarding. But first, you learn to pretend.

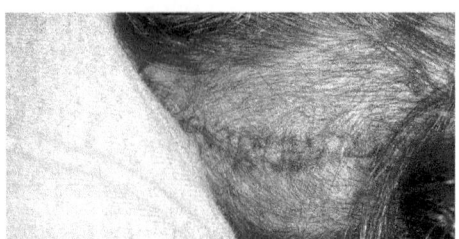

*Alessia's Decompression Incision, October 2016*
*Photo Credit: Stephanie Detjen Costabel*

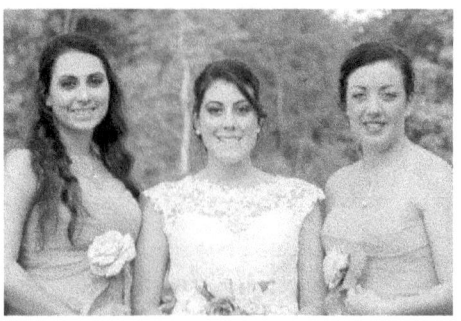

*Kassandra, Jatrin, and me at Jatrin's wedding, October 2016*
*All wedding Photo Credit: Jorge Gomez and Gerardo Londoño Photography*

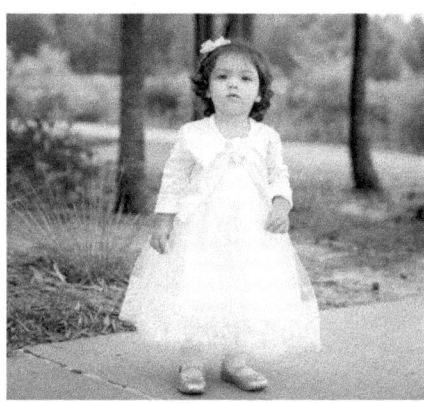

*Sophia at Jatrin's wedding, October 2016*

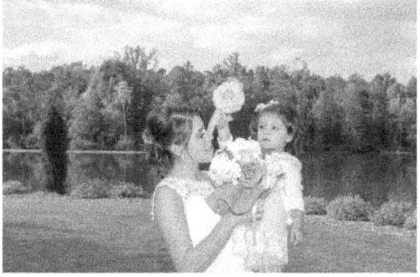

*Jatrin holding Sophia on her wedding day, October 2016*

## 15

I got nervous now when we had appointments with Dr. Daugherty. These last couple of appointments had been full of surprises and trips to the ER.

A week before Thanksgiving, we had our follow-up eye exam with him. It had been a month since her second decompression surgery, and he had to check her optic nerves to see that the swelling had gone down. As usual, I held my daughter down while Dr. D placed the eye opener speculum in her eyes. In my mind, I was begging for her optic nerves to be flat. But they weren't. The swelling had not gone down since her second decompression surgery.

Dr. D wanted to make sure that what he was seeing was papilledema, so he did an ultrasound on her eyes. "Her optic nerves appear elevated. Something is not right; they are still swollen. You should call Dr. Van Poppel and let him know. I'll call him too." He furrowed his eyebrows.

I shook my head. "I can't believe we are going through this again, Dr. D. What is going on?" I asked, fighting back the tears.

"I can't explain it," he replied. "She must have elevated ICP to cause her optic nerves to swell like this. Let's see what neurosurgery says."

"Do I have to rush her to the ER?"

"I think you need to call neurosurgery today. If they can see her this week, then I don't think going to the ER today is necessary." I nodded and left the appointment before I started to cry. On my way home, I made the phone call to neurosurgery and left a message for Dr. Van Poppel. They called me back within twenty minutes. Apparently, Dr. D had already made them aware of his findings, so they had already scheduled an MRI and CT scan with possible surgery the following morning at Levine's.

The rest of the afternoon I spent researching why Alessia's ICP could be so high. She had already had two decompression surgeries. There was not much else to do with her Chiari. I asked around in the RES and Chiari Facebook groups. Hydrocephalus and the need for a VP shunt was what most mothers informed me.

I knew that most kids with RES had hydrocephalus and it had been a concern that Alessia might end up developing hydrocephalus because of the size of her ventricles, but I was hoping we had passed that stage and her ventricles were stable after these decompression surgeries. Evidently something was wrong, and I had a feeling a VP shunt would be the next surgery she would end up having.

Later that evening, I sat on the living room couch and observed my girls. I had been so wrapped up in the surgeries and worries about Alessia's health that I realized I hadn't given Sophia much attention these last few months. She handed me a Minnie Mouse toy and looked up at me with large, happy eyes. She was getting so big. She was walking so well. I couldn't recall what day she had started walking. The guilt came rushing up my spine again—I swooped Sophia off her feet and hugged her tightly. My sweet Sophia. She had been a bystander throughout these last couple of months waiting patiently for me to give her the attention she needed. But Alessia always had my undivided attention. Because she was the sick one, she always needed me more.

But they all need me, I thought. How can I be such a terrible mother? I wish I could divide myself in three so each of my children can always have my undivided attention. A few minutes later, Sophia had fallen asleep in my arms. "I am going to sleep with you tonight, my dear," I whispered in her ear. I let Ronaldo handle Alessia's feeds and drifted off to sleep with Sophia. We needed that time together. I was most likely going to be gone the next two days for the MRI and possible shunt surgery, so it was Sophia's turn that night to have me all to herself.

They both were playing Ring Around the Rosie, holding hands and laughing together. The grass was a green fescue that looked like a carpet. There was nothing nearby—just miles and miles of grass. Both girls were barefoot, wearing white, fresh summer dresses. They were about five or six years old. They looked like angels. They both had long brown hair with golden highlights. They were identical. It was a warm, breezy, summer evening. The light bugs were starting to come out. "Tag, you're it!" Sophia said.

Alessia ran behind my legs. "It's not fair, Mommy, Sophia always tags me and I'm always it," she said, as a tear ran down her cheek.

"What do you mean? You are Sophia," I said, but then as I looked up, I saw Sophia standing there running away from us. I couldn't tell them apart. "Sophia, come here!" I yelled. "Don't go so far!"

"I'm Sophia, Mommy!" Alessia grabbed my shirt and pulled me to her. I was confused. They were playing jokes on me. They both were laughing at me and running down the green grass. They ran to a hill. I couldn't see what was on the other side of the hill . . .

"Wait, girls!" I yelled as I ran towards them. They kept running faster ahead of me. I couldn't keep up with them. They got to the top of the hill and suddenly I couldn't see Alessia. "Mommy! Come help!" Sophia screamed. "Alessia is drowning!"

My heart started racing as I ran as fast as I could to the hill. But the faster I ran, the farther the hill appeared. "Help, Mommy! Help!" Sophia sobbed. "She's dying, Mommy."

"Wake up. Baby, wake up!" I heard in the distance as I felt someone caressing my cheek. "It's time to go. It's already 7 a.m." Ronaldo kissed my cheek.

"Yes, yes, of course. I just had the weirdest dream with the girls." I yawned.

"Yeah, I could tell you were deep asleep—the alarm has been alarming for the last fifteen minutes." Ronaldo grinned down at me.

"The girls were both normal. They were playing and talking to each other. They were even joking and tricking me, they were identical. I couldn't tell them apart and then Alessia disappeared." I started crying.

"It's okay, babe. It was just a dream. It's too early for this, come on," he said as he helped me get up. He started getting Alessia's things ready.

"I wish you could go instead of me this time," I said as I got dressed. "I'm always the one that has to go to all these appointments and all these hospital stays." I had gotten up in a bad mood.

"You know I don't go because I don't understand absolutely everything that's going on with Alessia. You are the one that knows everything. You're the one that has done the research, and you are the one that will argue with the doctors if you need to. I wouldn't know what to do or what to say. She is in better hands with you than with me." He got closer to me and tucked a strand of my hair behind my ear.

"Yeah, I understand," I said as I got up and finished getting dressed. I was irritated. I was tired of being the only advocate for Alessia.

I arrived at Levine Children's Hospital, did the usual check-in process, and headed to the third floor: Radiology. After Pre-Op did its thing, I kissed my daughter goodbye. This time I didn't say a prayer.

After about two hours in the waiting room, they led me towards the same conference room we had been many times. Again. Dr. Van Poppel came in shortly after. "Hey there, I just finished reviewing Alessia's scans, and she is going to need a Ventriculoperitoneal shunt or VP shunt for short. She has hydrocephalus—her ventricles are large. I think it might be an absorption issue of CSF, so definitely needs a VP shunt. A VP shunt is a mechanical fix to the problem. We insert a thin plastic tube in her ventricles and run it to her stomach. This helps drain extra cerebral spinal fluid from the brain." He waited for my questions.

I didn't really have any questions for him. I had already read about hydrocephalus, VP shunts, and their high failure rate. "Will she always need one?" I raised an eyebrow.

"Right now, she does. If in the future she doesn't, then a shunt can always be removed. We'll go ahead and transfer her to the OR and get that done. I'll probably keep her overnight to observe her and get a repeat CT scan tomorrow morning. If everything goes well, you guys can go home tomorrow."

"Oh, that's not too bad. Much better than last time when we had to stay longer." I sighed.

"Well, a VP shunt placement is much less invasive than a decompression surgery, and since she did so well with her last surgeries, I don't anticipate any problems." He got up from his seat and left the room.

I stared out the window. I really hoped this was the last surgery they did to her developing brain. I knew it was a slim chance, since shunts have a high failure rate because they get clogged very easily, but I tried to be positive and hope we would all catch a break from this damn conference room. She needed a break. She had had back-to-back brain surgeries for the past three months.

I needed to blame somebody for Alessia's medical issues. But there really wasn't anybody to throw the blame at . . . except God, I thought. I couldn't dwell on that thought, though. Maybe God wasn't the blame here. Maybe there was no one to blame. Maybe shit just happens.

I often wonder what Alessia did to deserve this life. She had been through more than most of us go through in a lifetime. Surgery after surgery, incision after incision, she would always recover perfectly fine and act like nothing happened. She was so strong. We were discharged from the hospital a day after her VP shunt placement on November 23.

## 16

After Alessia's shunt surgery, we got a good break from the hospital. She didn't have any emergency surgeries or hospitalizations for a while. Alessia started developing at the speed of light. She started accepting a spoon and gained interest in food, although she would still cough occasionally if the spoon had too much food on it. But she would be able to safely swallow a few half-spoonfuls on a baby spoon. Her favorites were ice cream and smashed bananas with Nutella. This was not nearly enough to substitute a tube feeding, but at least she was getting the experience of taste. She would eat about half an ounce of ice cream or banana on a good day, and nothing on a bad day. I realized that I had gained more progress with her eating orally working with her at home at her own pace than during a whole year in feeding therapy. Alessia showed me that with time she would eat whenever she was ready and wanted to, not when I wanted her to. I didn't use a behavioral approach to her eating like the feeding clinic would. I let her take the lead and didn't make eating something she had to do.

I would offer her the spoon many times throughout the day while she played. If she opened her mouth, that meant she was interested in food. If she did not open her mouth, I would back away and respect her decision. I let her take control over her wants. It was the least I could do. There wasn't a whole lot she could control in her life. I wanted her to have the experience of taste and to be able to enjoy eating. My tactic worked because she slowly started eating. Little amounts of course but a lot more compared to when she was in feeding therapy.

Slowly but surely, she started walking. I had been warned by other mothers in the RES Facebook group that it was going to take time and she would fall a lot. They showed me different tactics on how to train her brain to catch herself when she fell. With Rhombencephalosynapsis, every unconscious movement your body made to protect itself—such as putting your arms out when you fall—had to be trained. It didn't come naturally to her. So, we worked endlessly with her physical therapist to train her brain to protect her body when she lost her balance. With a lot of hand-over-hand (holding her hand to guide her) and repetitive therapy she learned how to walk and catch herself when she fell. The PT brought a special walker for children who had balance issues, but Alessia never used it. She showed us early on she wasn't interested in any help.

By the summer, she was completely independent and walking all over the place. I was so proud. Her perseverance and determination to walk always triumphed over her fear of falling. Nothing ever scared her. Whereas other children would cry every time they fell, Alessia never seemed to mind falling or have much pain from falls. One time she fell so hard and scraped her knee so badly I thought I would have to take her to the hospital. But she didn't shed a tear. She got up and continued walking like nothing happened, even with blood dripping down her knee. She was so strong-willed, and it bothered her immensely to be helped. She would push us away every time we tried to help her get up from a fall. It was like she wanted to prove she could do it by herself. I had never met a child with so much strength and adaptability. Her disabilities never slowed her spirit.

Her personality started to flourish. She was independent and curious in her environment, but she rarely brought toys to me to play or interacted much with us. We really had to get in her face for her to notice us. Once she did notice us, she would smile and laugh. Sometimes we got the impression she was ignoring us on purpose. She was attracted to the weirdest things: lights, anything shiny or colorful, pieces of yarn, texturized and patterned objects, sand, water . . . she craved sensory stimulation. I would notice her staring and touching the patterns of our granite countertops, or the grout lines from our floor tiles.

For their second birthday, I had a party at the park with an Easter egg hunt, since Easter was around the corner. She never noticed the Easter eggs or the people around her. She was content with feeling the grass or pine needles or staring at the sunlight reflecting from the silver lining on the slide. She was obsessed with Mardi Gras beads and shiny necklaces, but she wouldn't put them on. She would hold them up and watch them dangle from her hand. She did not like to sit still, and if she did, she needed to be fixated on a certain object, whether it be a dangling bead or a sensory toy. But if she was not entertained by something sensory, she would constantly be on the move looking for sensory input.

We started her in auditory verbal therapy to hopefully get her to develop speech. She was two and a half years old and had no words yet. At first, she showed interest in various light-up toys with the therapist. We would sing the "Itsy Bitsy Spider" song and try to get her to sing along with us or at least make the noise of the tune. She did it a couple of times, but after a few weeks she started to regress. It was around the end of the summer. She did not want to sit in her seat or participate in the therapies. We tried sign language with her, but she showed no interest.

I wasn't quite sure if it was that she did not have any interest in signing, or if she could not coordinate her fingers and hands to do the sign that was being taught to her. What I did know was that she did not like to be pressured or forced to do something she did not want to do. She hated being strapped in a chair. She showed us early on that if she was not interested, she would not pay attention no matter how hard we tried. She was stubborn: her way or no way on the highway. But her stubbornness was the fuel she needed to develop and independently problem-solve. She didn't need us. Slowly, but surely, she would figure things out.

Towards the end of the summer when she was uncomfortable, she would want to be held and swayed back and forth. I couldn't really differentiate whether it was pain or just the frustration of not being able to communicate. But it seemed her only relief to whatever was bothering her. At first it was every so often, but then it became a daily thing.

We went twice that year to the beach, which she loved. The sensory input she received from the sand and the waves was medicine to her. I had never seen her so happy as when she was at the beach. She was a free spirit . . . wild . . . independent . . . figuring the world out on her own. We didn't need to figure out the world out for her. She showed us she was perfectly capable of figuring it out herself. It wasn't her disabilities that slowed her down, it was the discomfort of her body that made life difficult for her.

We bought a house that year: a beautiful, 3,000-square-foot house with a nice fenced-in leveled backyard. We had rented up until that point, so it felt great to have a house of our own, as well as so much space. Alessia loved exploring the new house. She had a lot of places to go and wander.

Around the end of summer, Alessia would have these raging outbursts and cry uncontrollably. I couldn't figure out a specific trigger. It seemed to happen out of nowhere. She started dragging her head again and doing headstands and poking her eyes. It was extremely frustrating and confusing. Some days she would laugh while poking her eyes or cry uncontrollably until I picked her up and swayed her back and forth. Other days she didn't want to be touched. She would slap her head and pull her hair. The frustration of not being able to communicate when something was wrong is what most of her therapists and specialists suggested as to why she was so upset.

I needed her to tell me what was wrong or at least point to what hurt, but no matter how hard I tried to get her to communicate she just could not. I had her on a feeding schedule with her tube feedings and water flushes, but she could not tell me if she was thirsty or if she was hungry, or if I had given her too much food and her tummy hurt. Or if she had gas or needed to poop. It became a habit for her to melt down and poke her eyes every time she needed something or felt off. It was her relief to go for her eyes constantly.

Because of this, we dealt with many corneal abrasions and ulcers. Thankfully, all of them that year healed. I needed to stop the behavior somehow, but I was lost as to why exactly she poked her eyes. I posted a video on the RES Facebook group of Alessia having meltdowns and eye poking to see if there was another parent who had any solution. That's when I met Page, another mom whose son had RES and GLHS who had the same constant eye poking behaviors. Her little boy had Chiari but still had not been decompressed, and she attributed a lot of his eye poking behaviors to pain: head pain to be exact. The way she explained it to me was that since these kids have corneal anesthesia (meaning they cannot feel the surface of the eye), they dig into their eyes, trying to get to the source of the pain/discomfort. They could feel internal pain, just not corneal pain.

When you have a headache, you press on your temples or in between your eyes to try to alleviate the pain. The pressure of your fingers often helps. RES kiddos with corneal anesthesia do not feel the pressure of their fingers until they are deep inside the eye. I started alternating Motrin and Tylenol to see if it would help with the discomfort. It did seem to alleviate some, and the eye poking decreased a little. But everything caused her head pain. If she had gas, if she was constipated, if it was a rainy day and the barometric pressure of the atmosphere was high, if she had allergies or a cold or a sinus infection or tooth pain . . . Everything uncomfortable triggered eye poking.

Trips to see Dr. D. became a weekly thing, and eye ointment and eye drops were a daily thing. Sometimes we even had to use arm restraints. Anything to protect her corneas. But Alessia was so smart and stubborn, she would always find a way to remove her arm restraints. If she couldn't poke her eye with her fingers, she would use her toes. Every day I would treat anything that could possibly cause her discomfort. I would start with gas drops, Miralax, suppositories, Motrin, Tylenol, Zyrtec, more water, less water, more food, less food. It was a guessing game.

We saw Dr. Van Poppel a couple of times throughout the summer and ran CT scans and MRIs to make sure her shunt was okay. He referred us to a neurologist for migraine management. We tried cyproheptadine, gabapentin, propranolol, and even narcotics when we felt the other meds did not help.

Meanwhile, in auditory verbal therapy, she would fight every time she was seated in an upright position. She would cry, melt down, and eye poke until we let her out. She always wanted to rest her head on the table or on the floor. She would not respond consistently to sounds.

Another sedated BAER hearing test was ordered, this time at UNC Chapel Hill since they were the best of the best for hearing impairment. We saw an ENT there as well, who ordered a sedated CT scan of her inner ears to see if she would potentially be a candidate for cochlear implants.

It was a hot, summer day when we drove to Raleigh to get her tests done. She had to be under anesthesia, so we gave her the last feeding the night before. This was the first time she would go under anesthesia in Chapel Hill, so I was a little nervous. Thankfully, everything went well.

The results of her CT scans and BAER hearing test showed her inner ears were malformed. Her cochlea on both sides did not develop the way they were supposed to. A normal cochlea has two and a half turns, but hers only had a little more than half. Known as Cochlear Hypoplasia, this disorder would cause a reverse slope hearing loss, so she would hear higher frequencies more than lower frequencies. High pitch tunes like the voice of a child or consonants were heard by her. But Alessia could not hear vowels and low pitch sounds. Whereas a normal child could pick up the word "Mama," Alessia could only pick up "M, M." The situation would make it more difficult for her to learn how to speak.

The malformation of the cochlea and the fact she had a shunt running down the side of her head made a cochlear implant extremely difficult to do surgically. The best option for her was to continue using her BAHA on a soft band to allow her to pick up the little sound she could.

We shifted from auditory verbal therapy to try to teach her sign language. I would repeat signs such as "more" or "eat" fifty million times throughout the day. Hand over hand with repetitive motions, every time I would feed her, I would show her the sign for "eat." Every time she wanted something, whether it was a shiny bead necklace or for me to pick her up and sway her, I would repeat hand over hand the sign for "up" or "more." I spent hours daily, repeating signs, showing her how to make them with her tiny hands. No matter how hard I tried, she would just not pick it up. I grew exhausted. It was like feeding therapy; no matter how many times I would offer her the spoon, some days she just would not cooperate. The difference was that with feeding she would sometimes want a taste of ice cream. With sign language, she never wanted to mimic a sign or showed any interest in communicating. I never pressured her, but I did show the signs repeatedly in her face, hoping she would one day show interest.

I learned some sign language and taught it to Thiago and Sophia to start communicating in sign language to see if Alessia would catch on.

She didn't pay any attention. She was always in her own little world, interested in things most of us would have no interest in.

She did have some good days where her interaction with us amazed me. One day I was singing "Ring Around the Rosie" to both girls, and she started twirling around and trying to hold Sophia's hands. I thought she might have heard me and wanted to play along. She did that a couple of times . . . but then she would regress and not do it anymore. There were also a couple of days where she said, "mamamama," not necessarily calling me, but just vocalizing and babbling. I would get super excited when she would do those things and thought she was starting to make progress, but then she wouldn't repeat it for weeks. She would take one step forward and ten steps back.

On her good days, we enjoyed being a normal family. We went to a farm one day and saw farm animals and went to a pumpkin patch. I thought she would be interested in the animals, but she didn't really notice them. For Halloween, the girls dressed up as Peppa Pig and Thiago as an Enderman from Minecraft. It was hard work to prepare all of Alessia's feeds and make sure she didn't wander off during our outings, but no matter how difficult it was to go out and do normal things, we still tried. I have pictures to look back on to remind me that not everything was so grim all the time. Even if Alessia did not notice that she had a costume on for Halloween. Even if she had no idea who Peppa Pig was and didn't care to trick-or-treat, I still took pictures of her with the candy. She didn't even taste them, but she would have fun with the wrappers.

November was time for Alessia's post-op six-month checkup—a rapid sequence MRI, basically a limited sequence MRI protocol that eliminates ionizing radiation exposure and reduces imaging time. It was good that she did not have to be sedated for it and it was done at the Carolina Neurosurgery and Spine Associates, not at the hospital. That was good for me since by that point I had major PTSD from being at the hospital.

I had to go with Alessia in the MRI tube and hold her head still while they took the pictures. Alessia did very well.

Dr. Van Poppel would call us in a few days to go over the results.

My sisters came home for Thanksgiving. My mother and her boyfriend, Sam, came over as well. My mother made a delicious turkey that we ate heartily. The sweet potato casserole, asparagus pie, homemade mac and cheese, and mashed potatoes were breathtakingly good. By the end of the day, we were stuffed from so much eating. It was so nice to spend Thanksgiving Day with the whole family. Alessia seemed calm throughout most of the evening; however, towards the end of the night we realized she was uncomfortable. She would stand and strain. It was obvious she was trying to defecate. She was severely constipated, and it was hurting her. My sister, who is a nurse, looked at her bottom and could see she was impacted. She put gloves on and helped the impaction come out. Once all the stool came out, Alessia was in a much better mood. In the midst of Thanksgiving, I felt so sorry for her. My poor Alessia . . . she can't eat orally, she can't hear, she can't talk, and now she can't even poop on her own. How do you calm the constant worrying about the well-being of your child?

A couple of weeks after Thanksgiving, I was surprised to receive a call from Carolina Neurosurgery and Spine Associates. They had called me a few weeks before to assure me her scans looked fine and there was no need to adjust her shunt settings.

"Hi, Mrs. Costabel! How are you?" It was Dr. Van Poppel's physician assistant, Lauren. I recognized her voice.

"I'm doing pretty good. How about yourself? What's up?" I asked. They usually never called like this, and my heart started racing. "Dr. Van Poppel has reviewed the latest scan and we need to adjust her shunt. Her ventricles are small . . . very close to being considered slit ventricles. We need to lower her settings, so she has less CSF drainage and hopefully plump up her ventricles a little bit."

"Yes, of course," I replied. "Can I go later today?" I asked nervously.

"Yes, I'll see you later this afternoon," she replied.

Slit ventricle syndrome. Finally, an answer to her head pain? Why did they say everything was fine a few weeks before?

Slit ventricle syndrome is caused by an over-draining shunt. It can cause excruciating headaches that are only relieved when lying down. This made sense since Alessia was constantly lying to her side and putting her head down. This must be the reason for her discomfort, I thought. I quickly got the girls ready and headed to Carolina Neurosurgery and Spine Associates. We needed to get this shunt adjusted ASAP.

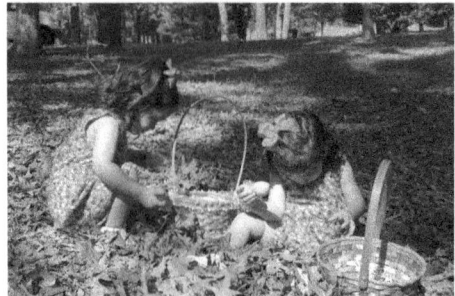 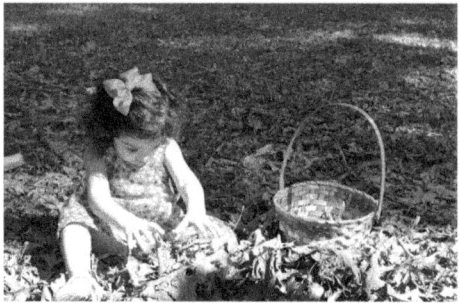

*2017 Photo Credit: Stephanie Detjen Costabel*

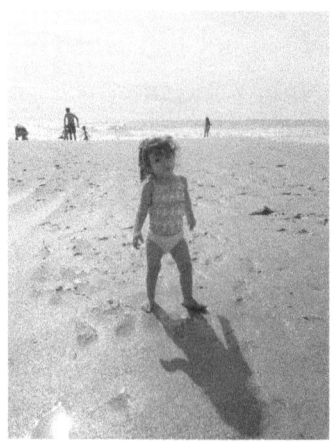 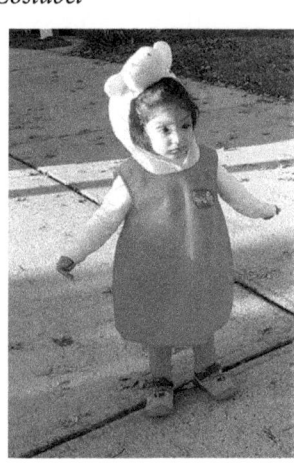

*Alessia as Peppa Pig Halloween, 2017 Photo Credit: Stephanie Detjen Costabel*

## 17

Alessia's VP shunt was adjusted to 2.5. On this setting, the least amount of cerebral spinal fluid was drained from her ventricles. Dr. Van Poppel thought it would help her ventricles puff up a bit. A few days after this adjustment, she made a 180-degree turn in her mood. She was laughing most of the day and overall, quite happy. She seemed to not have much pain and the eye poking behavior decreased dramatically. She was paying more attention to us. I was encouraged.

Christmas was so much fun for the whole family. Alessia even danced to the music and helped open the presents. It's amazing how awesome life is when your medically complex child is happy. The things people take for granted: good health by far being the most important, in my opinion.

I was in so many Facebook groups. Each one was dedicated to Alessia's separate illnesses and symptoms: feeding tube weaning, RES, Chiari, hydrocephalus, special needs, hearing impairment, tracheolaryngo-malacia, alternative medicine, and at one point cannabis oil therapy. I realized that the best advice came from other parents that dealt with similar issues. I was willing to try anything. Anything that could possibly improve her quality of life.

I had heard good things about Charlotte's Web CBD oil. I had heard from other moms in Facebook groups dedicated to special-needs kids that it could help with her mood and pain. I started her on a few drops, and whether it was the reprogramming of her shunt to 2.5 or the CBD oil, I did not know, but Alessia was the happiest she had ever been.

That's why it caught me by utter surprise when we went to check her optic nerves in March of that year and Dr. D discovered she had bilateral papilledema. Again . . .

"It's impossible—it can't be! Look at her! Look at her joy! She can't have papilledema! If she had elevated ICP she wouldn't feel this way!" I yelled.

"I'm sorry," Dr. D said. I could tell he was worried. "Her optic nerves are elevated. You must let neurosurgery know. Maybe they can check her shunt and make sure it's working properly. I strongly recommend you call Dr. Van Poppel. I'm sorry."

I nodded and held back my tears. I just could not think of her having to endure another surgery, especially when Alessia was doing so well.

I called CSNA on my way back home. "Hi, I need to leave a message for Dr. Van Poppel, please, regarding Alessia Cruz."

"Dr. Van Poppel is out of the country. He won't be back in clinic until later next week," the receptionist said.

*Damn. Now what do I do?* "Is there any other provider that is taking over his patients?" I asked.

"Dr. Wate is taking over his caseload while he is gone. I can schedule you in for an appointment with him on Monday morning if you'd like."

Monday was six days away, but I figured it would be fine since she was doing so well. If it were a true shunt malfunction, she would be lethargic and throwing up. Something was definitely wrong with her shunt to cause papilledema or her Chiari . . . please don't let it be the Chiari.

"Yes, please schedule me for Monday morning with Dr. Wate."

After I hung up with CSNA I called Dr. D's office to make sure he sent over his findings from the eye exam over to them. I figured that if they had actual proof from another specialist of her papilledema, they would do a quick lumbar puncture to check her opening pressure and we would know if Alessia's shunt was malfunctioning.

Monday morning came around and we met with Dr. Wate. Most neurosurgeons seem to have a peculiar personality. They go through so much schooling to become brain surgeons that I feel it takes a toll on their personality, or at least with their patients. Dr. Wate wasn't dismissive or arrogant in any way, just not very talkative, just like Dr. Van Poppel. They go straight to the point and sometimes won't explain things in detail the way I would like it to be explained to me. I want to know everything. Even if I don't understand it.

"We will need to do ICP monitoring on Alessia," Dr. Wate said.

"What exactly is ICP monitoring and why do we need to do it? Can't we just do a lumbar puncture?" I asked.

"A lumbar puncture won't give us accurate ICP results. ICP monitoring will give us an idea of what her ICP pressure does during the day and night. She doesn't have the classic symptoms of shunt malfunction. She has papilledema only and I'm not exactly sure if her shunt is entirely malfunctioning. So, basically, we insert a bolt with a tiny sensor into her ventricles and measure it for a few days. Twenty-four to fifty-eight hours approximately."

I could feel shivers go down my spine. "So, is this a surgery? Explain to me how you insert the bolt." I started feeling sick to my stomach.

"We drill a small hole in her skull to be able to insert her sensor into her ventricles," he replied.

Oh my God, are you serious? I thought. My heart skipped a beat.

"It's not that invasive," he said. "It's a very small hole just to be able to put the sensor in. She needs to be monitored closely since she will be connected to the ICP monitor. She can't be pulling at it. That's why she needs to stay in the hospital while the bolt is in. At the end of the ICP monitoring, we should have a good idea if her shunt is malfunctioning and if it is, we will remove the bolt and do a shunt revision under anesthesia."

"When is Dr. Van Poppel coming back?" I asked.

"He will be here on Thursday, so if you would like we can do the ICP procedure on Wednesday. That way on Thursday when Dr. Van Poppel is here, he can decide what needs to be done." He got up to exit the room.

I really couldn't complain. She had been out of the hospital for a long time and was doing relatively well. The vomiting had stopped and her desaturations at night had stopped. She wasn't requiring oxygen at night. I guess when you have a medically complex child, every once in a while, you do have to go back to the hospital for some test or procedure. Is this really how it's going to be all her life? We should really enjoy the time we are not in a hospital, I thought.

"I'll have the scheduler call you and let you know your arrival time." He smiled and quickly exited the room.

I'd become terrified of staying in the hospital and hated staying there. I hated that Alessia had to go through yet another medical procedure to figure out what was wrong. It was a never-ending battle. In the twenty-first century, how was there not another less invasive way to check if her shunt was working well?

Ronaldo was waiting for me in the front porch when I pulled into the driveway. "So, what happened? What did they say?" he asked nervously.

"Hi, how are you? would have been nice." I rolled my eyes at him. The stress of having a medically complex child definitely takes a toll on your marriage. I explained to him what was happening, while avoiding making eye contact with him. He was obviously upset at the news and didn't say much for the rest of the day. It killed me inside to not have anyone to really talk to about Alessia that would understand the struggles we faced. Not only with her, but our whole family in general. Everyone suffers. Our marriage suffered. Our other children suffered.

## An Amazing Little Girl with Rhombencephalosynapsis

Wednesday morning came and we knew the drill. We were led to pre-op and they did the usual pre-op procedure. I kissed Alessia on her soft cheek and was led to the same waiting room. I was so used to surgeries that it surprised me that I didn't get nervous anymore. An hour later, she was done, and the ICP bolt had been inserted. Now we just had to get the data and figure out what was wrong with her shunt. I was led to the PICU and Alessia was already starting to wake up. The poor thing looked like a unicorn. The bolt stuck out of the top of her forehead. I gasped at the thought she could easily pull it out. But to my surprise she didn't seem to mind it.

"What was her opening ICP pressure?" I asked the nurse as I laid my backpack on the chair.

"It was 15, which is pretty normal, but she was under anesthesia, so we won't get accurate results until later tonight or tomorrow." She started administering antibiotic and pain meds through her IV.

The rest of the night Alessia was pretty much out of it from the anesthesia. I, on the other hand, was like a hawk watching her ICP monitor. 15, 20, 30, then back down to 10. Her ICP seemed to go all over the place. I repositioned her throughout the night to see if her position affected her ICP numbers, but I couldn't tell. I googled all night about ICP. Evidently it was elevated. Normal ranges are from 5 to about 10. Alessia's ranged from 5 all the way up to mid-20s and 30s. I can't recall exactly at what time I fell asleep that night, but it was sometime after 2 a.m. I should have just chilled out and let the doctors/nurses do their job. But I was always trying to be ahead of the game. Always researching and reading about Alessia's medical problems. This was a good thing but also a bad thing. Good because I will always be Alessia's best advocate, and an informed mother is a good mother. Bad because you can stress the living shit out of yourself with all that researching that you miss out on actually being a normal mom.

I woke up to Alessia babbling. God forbid she yanks that bolt out, I thought. I quickly jumped into her hospital bed and lay with her. She was in a good mood. Funny, after all she had been through.

The doctors usually round around 10 a.m., and it was only 7 a.m.

"Any events in particular that raised your eyebrows?" I asked the nurse when she walked in to give Alessia her meds. God, I could have at least said good morning. I was in such a crappy mood.

"Well, you will have to wait till Dr. Wate rounds, but her ICP has been pretty stable."

I went to get some coffee. I needed to be alert for when Dr. Wate came to do rounds.

They came to round, and it was Dr. Wate's physician assistant instead of Dr. Wate. I hated when this happened: not that the physician assistants can't give me an update, but I have always preferred to talk directly with Alessia's doctors.

"Good morning." Dr. Wate's PA greeted me with a smile from ear to ear. She seemed to have a bubbly personality, which I appreciated.

"So, what have you discovered with her ICP and what is the plan?" I asked abruptly. I probably should have been nicer, but I was so exhausted and tired that I could not be nice to anyone at that point.

"Her ICP is elevated. We are going to adjust her shunt to see if it helps. We are going to put it on a higher setting, so more cerebral spinal fluid will flow out of her shunt. If her ICP decreases, then she just needs a change of setting. If the ICP remains high, then that's a clear indication her shunt is malfunctioning."

Reprogramming a shunt is a relatively simple procedure. With a magnet they can adjust the shunt to have more fluid or less fluid flow. The PA got out her magnet to adjust the shunt, then said, "It will take a few hours to see any difference. By tomorrow morning we will have a better idea as to what's going on—Dr. Van Poppel will be here tomorrow, and you can discuss your options with him."

I nodded. Twenty-four more hours to know what the damn problem was. "I do want to ask you about her Chiari and if it could have anything to do with it. Also Slit Ventricle Syndrome? Talk to me about that, please. Since her ventricles are so tiny and close to slit-like. Could that also explain the headaches she gets sometimes?" I asked.

"So, Alessia's ventricles are small, but they are not considered slit-like ventricles, yet. If you stay with Slit Ventricle Syndrome for a very long time then this can cause headaches. But it usually takes years. I doubt she is having headaches from slit-like ventricles."

I wasn't understanding much. I should have studied neurosurgery.

That second night, I couldn't stop researching and reading about Hydrocephalus, ICP, and Slit Ventricle Syndrome. Thankfully, Alessia had fallen asleep early, so I took advantage and read every single medical article on slit vents. I wanted to know everything about the brain and how it works. I just couldn't understand how it took years to have headaches due to Slit Ventricle Syndrome. Alessia's shunt was adjusted back in November because she was close to slit-like vents, and her mood improved, the headstands stopped, and her irritability decreased; but on the other hand, I couldn't understand how she could look so well and yet have elevated ICP pressures. I soon drifted off to sleep.

I was awakened by a familiar voice.

It was Dr. Van Poppel talking to the night shift nurse. I quickly got up. "Oh my God, I'm so incredibly happy and relieved to see you!"

"Good morning! So, I've reviewed Alessia's ICP numbers throughout these last forty-eight hours. Something is definitely wrong, but I'm not entirely sure what it is. I think we need to do an exploratory surgery to see if her shunt is working properly." He scratched his beard, looking concerned.

"Exploratory surgery? What are your thoughts exactly? Do you think it's the shunt? If it isn't the shunt, then what can it be? Do you think it might be the Chiari?"

"I did a pretty big decompression surgery, so I don't think it's her Chiari. I think it's something in her shunt, but I am not 100 percent sure, so that's why I want to go ahead and do exploratory surgery to actually see her shunt."

"Okay, but what if you explore the shunt and it's not it?" I asked. I was being annoying.

"Well, if her shunt is fine then we would be talking about a bigger surgery. Craniosynostosis. I don't think we need to get into that conversation right now. Let's explore her shunt and go from there. You haven't given her any food this morning, right?" he asked.

"No, I haven't fed her yet." I tried to calm down to not bombard him with any more questions.

"Okay, good. Pre-op will be here soon to do their part and I will see her in the OR at 10 a.m." He exited the room.

The term "exploratory surgery" is what got to me. The not knowing. This uncertainty is what drives you crazy.

After Pre-op did its job, she was ready to go. I whispered in Alessia's ear, "I love you." I don't know if she heard me or not, but she squeezed my finger. I always cried when they wheeled her bed back to the OR. God, I hate this feeling.

Two hours later, Dr. Van Poppel had completed the surgery. I met him in the conference room, biting my nails.

"She is doing well. Everything is fine now. Her shunt catheter was partially clogged with scar tissue. I replaced the catheter and made sure the cerebral spinal fluid flowed freely. Her shunt is working fine now. I want to keep her overnight and have another CT scan in the morning. If everything looks well, you guys should be able to go home tomorrow afternoon."

I sighed. I was so relieved. All that reading and researching the "what ifs?" All it did was stress the hell out of me. But I was fine now. Now we just needed to go home and go on with our lives, or at least I hoped.

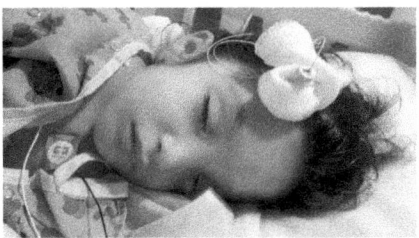

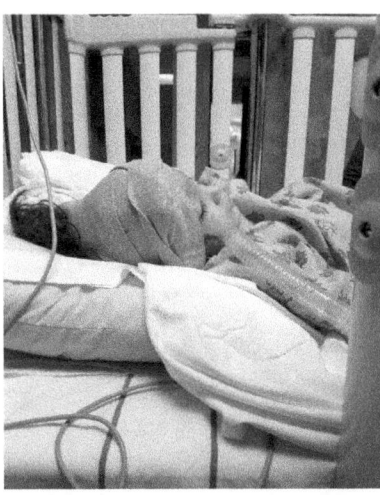

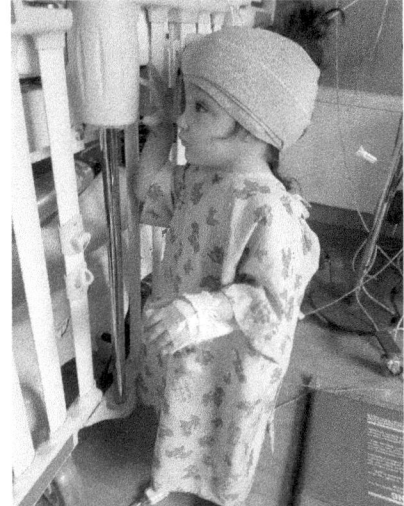

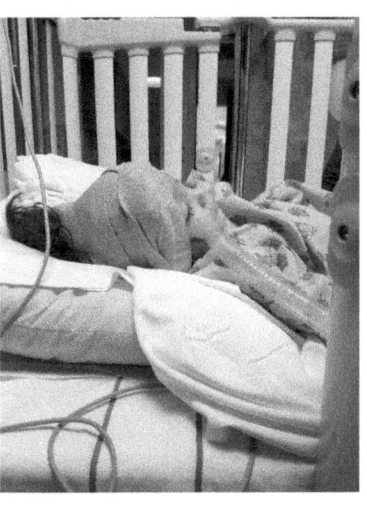

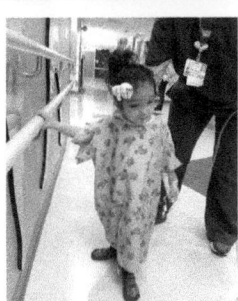

*Alessia's ICP monitoring and shunt revision, March 2017*
*Photo Credit: Stephanie Detjen Costabel*

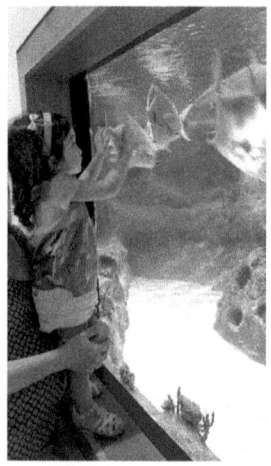
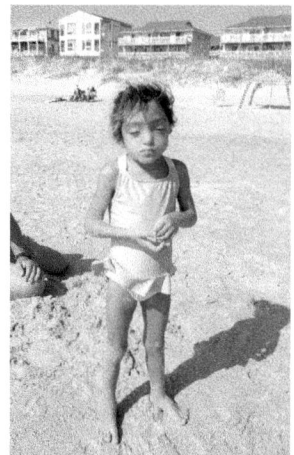
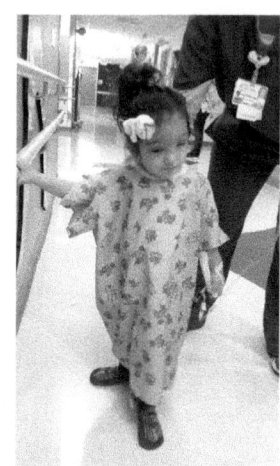
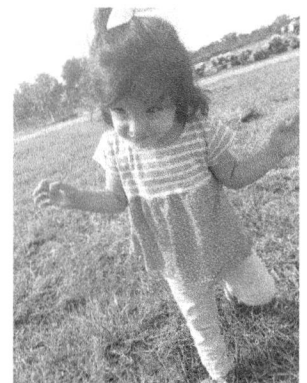
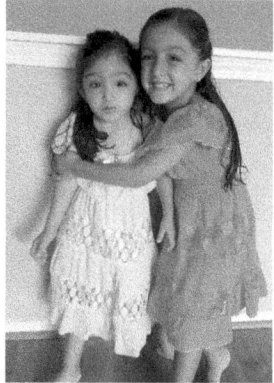

*2017 Moments*
*Photo Credit: Stephanie Detjen Costabel*

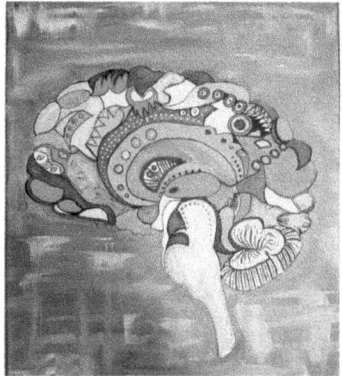

*An abstract brain I painted in appreciation for Dr. Van Poppel, 2017*
*Photo Credit: Stephanie Detjen Costabel*

# 18

The night we came home I slept fifteen hours straight. All that stress of worrying and researching and trying to be one step ahead of the game caught up to me, not to mention the comfort of being at home and sleeping in my own bed. I loved my bed. I loved being home. Alessia slept for twelve hours straight.

I had missed Sophia and Thiago and they'd missed me. Sophia was more clingy than usual, and Thiago wouldn't stop talking about all that he had done in the past two days while I was gone. Anyone would think I'd been gone for a year!

That night in bed, as I smelled the crisp clean sheets of my pillow, I began questioning my worries. Time and time again Alessia proved to me she was willing to fight the battle and live. *Why am I so paranoid about losing her? Why do I question every single decision we made with her doctors? Why do I not trust anyone with my daughter's care? We are home now, sleeping in our beds, and we are fine.* I had to learn to trust in Alessia's specialists. But how could I when I always felt on edge when it came to Alessia's health?

Alessia did relatively well for a while, but by the summer of 2018, she was back at it again with her irritability, headstands, and headaches. For a child who is deaf and nonverbal, the only way we could understand what she was feeling was by observing her behaviors. I sought out help from her doctors—GI, pulmonology, neurology, and even the ENT. We put tubes in her only ear because the ENT saw she had fluid behind her ear drum and that surely it was causing her discomfort. After the ear tube surgery, and after GI did a thorough evaluation on her GI tract, we tried probiotics and gabapentin for nerve pain. We tried everything. We found a developmental pediatrician who diagnosed her with level two autism and prescribed her Applied Behavioral Analysis (ABA) therapy. But there was nothing that could explain her irritability and self-injurious behaviors.

Applied Behavioral Analysis therapy applies to our understanding of how behavior works in real situations. The goal is to increase behaviors that are helpful and decrease behaviors that are harmful or affect learning. The way it works involves different teaching tactics. Positive reinforcement is one of the main strategies used in ABA.

When a behavior is followed by something that is valued (a reward), a person is more likely to repeat that behavior. Over time, this encourages positive behavior change. First, the therapist identifies a goal behavior. Each time the person uses the behavior or skill successfully, they get a reward. The reward is meaningful to the individual—examples include praise, a toy or book, watching a video, access to playground or other location, and more.

Positive rewards encourage the person to continue using the skill. Over time, this leads to meaningful behavior change. When the individual expresses negative behaviors such as self-injurious behaviors or behaviors not acceptable in today's society, the therapist tries to discourage this behavior by removing eye contact and ignoring the child that is doing these unacceptable behaviors. ABA therapy is focused to train the individual to act appropriately in a normal social setting. So basically, they are trained to act a specific way to either get a reward if they do what is expected of them, or a punishment, which in most cases consisted of ignoring their self-injurious behaviors to get them to not do them.

ABA therapy is controversial. I had heard the good and the bad, but I decided I was going to give it a try. None of her specialists had any medical explanations to her behaviors, so they all thought it most likely was behavioral and she just needed ABA therapy.

Two months after we got on the waiting list, she started. Different therapists came to my house for eight hours each day and repeated the same behavior expectation, over and over again. They tried to train Alessia to behave in a way that was appropriate. This might work for a child who is not medically complex and only autistic. But for a child who is medically complex, deaf, and autistic, this therapy proved to be a failure at the time. She wasn't learning anything from it, and I hated the sessions. The more I observed the ABA therapy sessions with my daughter, the more convinced I was that her behaviors were coming from some deep eye or head pain, not behavioral meltdowns. I soon realized that the ABA therapists working with Alessia were not trained to interact with hearing-impaired children. ABA therapists use the Picture Exchange System, known as PECS, to try to get a child to communicate by using pictures. Many times, I observed our ABA therapist working with Alessia and asking her to point at the picture that represented an apple. But the therapist would put the pictures in front of her mouth. How could Alessia point to what the therapist was requesting when she couldn't hear her? She had no way of relating the picture to the verbal word. No matter how many times I asked for them to use signs, they would use them for the first few hours and then forget and go back to verbal demands. It was extremely difficult for me to watch these ABA therapy sessions and not get frustrated.

There was one ABA session where Alessia wanted to get on the trampoline. Her way of communicating was to pull you and put your hand to whatever it was she wanted. If you didn't do it, she would melt down. When Alessia pulled the therapist's hand on the trampoline, the therapist said, "No," and Alessia started melting down. The ABA therapist removed eye contact from her and ignored her while she had a meltdown.

A tear ran down my cheek as I watched from the window. I can understand ignoring bad behavior in a normal developing child who is just having a tantrum. But Alessia was nonverbal and hearing-impaired, as well as medically complex. Her brain was malformed. It wasn't that she refused to speak, it was that she just couldn't. For her to be able to communicate using her hands was huge. I suppose she could not coordinate her fingers to make signs because of her brain abnormalities. Maybe she wouldn't speak because she could not open half of her mouth all the way and move her tongue to be able to create language. She was frustrated because she was not being understood. When she tried to be understood with her gestures, as a team we needed to encourage it. We needed to reward it. So, if Alessia used her hands to signal that she wants something, we should honor it. We should encourage it. Not just say, "No," and ignore her meltdown from frustration.

By the end of the summer, I knew that ABA therapy was not a good fit for Alessia.

During the summer, I went back to Neurosurgery and asked for another Chiari protocol MRI. We had tried adjusting her shunt many times, and she was still doing the headstands and eye poking and was overall miserable.

On August 26, 2018, Alessia went in for a sedated Chiari protocol MRI and CINE study. Afterwards we met with Dr. Van Poppel to go over the results.

"Everything looks good." Dr. Van Poppel said. "She has good CSF flow. Nothing that really could explain headaches, so you will have to consult with neurology about migraine management."

I pressed my lips together. One part of me was scared that there was something in her brain that was causing her headaches and we would have to do yet another brain surgery to resolve it. Another part of me wished they would have found something on the MRI that could explain her headaches so we would have a solution to her pain and behaviors. I thanked Dr. Van Poppel, picked Alessia up, and headed out the door.

Another dead-end.

We had already tried medication and it hadn't helped. Something was missing, something was not right.

That same night, I decided to pull up the images from her MRI from that day. I had never looked at any of Alessia's scans from the past. Mainly because I did not have much knowledge about the anatomy of the brain, so I wasn't going to be able to understand what I was seeing. I had gotten close to Deanna from the RES Facebook page. We messaged each other often and she had a lot of knowledge about the brain and Chiari. She had been extremely helpful when it came to Alessia's diagnosis the first time, so surely, she would be able to help me understand the images.

Deanna was willing to help me interpret the results of the MRI in a way I could understand. It was helpful to have another mom of an RESer who would take the time to explain things in detail. I inserted the MRI CD on my laptop and there were over 170 images. I had absolutely no idea what I was looking at.

"I do not know which one to look at," I messaged Deanna.

"It will be the image closest to the middle. So, if there are a total of 170 images, it should be around image 85 or 86, that's the one that's going to give you the clearest view," she replied.

I forwarded through all the images and got to number 87. That gave me the clearest axial view of Alessia's brain. I screenshotted the image and messaged it to Deanna. While I was waiting for her to reply, I googled pictures of the anatomy of a normal three-year-old child's brain. Alessia's brain looked totally different. The cerebellum appeared incredibly low, almost to her neck. The brainstem did not appear straight like it appeared in a normal brain. Everything in that image I saw looked abnormal. My heart started racing and my hands trembled as I waited for Deanna to reply. She wasn't a neurosurgeon, but she was knowledgeable. She had always been right, even when it came to Alessia's first Chiari diagnosis. I had never met her nor talked to her on the phone, but something about her expertise on the matter made me trust in her. My breathing became fast as I waited for her reply. After a couple minutes, it finally came through.

"Holy crap."

I read those two words and suddenly my heart sank.

"Two things . . . " She had drawn an arrow pointing to her Chiari on the image I had sent her. "First, she is still super pinched there. Do you see that? It's like her cerebellum tonsil is pinched off in the spinal canal—almost folded in half. Second, she has bone pushing into her freaking brainstem. Does she look at the ground ever? Like chin down? Because I would worry that would kill her. Maybe not literally, but definitely pain."

My vision became blurry as I kept reading Deanna's incoming messages. "That is a super touchy area of the brain, and it is not supposed to be folded over bone and I suddenly don't like your surgeon for decompressing her to the point of cerebellar slumping without touching that. I'm out of my depth. We have no personal experience with it, but I think they can try a cervical collar to lift the neck. Or surgery. What that surgery entails, I do not know, but I would see Dr. Greenfield or Dr. Grant. If your current neurosurgeon says she has no reason to hurt and it's normal, that's your answer on pursuing care there. Google 'Basilar Invagination.' It can hurt."

# An Amazing Little Girl with Rhombencephalosynapsis

*Basilar invagination: periods of confusion. Difficulty swallowing or saying words due to loss of muscle control. Dizziness. Loss of sensation. Pain in the back of the head. Tingling or numbness in the 4th and 5th fingers. Tingling when the neck bends forward or backward. Weakness or stiff awkward movements of the arms and legs.* Could this be it? I did not get any sleep that night.

As soon as the clock hit 8 a.m., I called Carolina Neurosurgery and Spine Associates, furious.

"Mrs. Costabel, I have looked at the scans and everything looks fine compared to the one two years ago. After decompression, some slumping is expected."

"No, it hasn't!" I scolded the P.A. over the phone. "She did not have basilar invagination and look at how low her cerebellum is! She has cerebellar slumping! All this causes pain! How can you guys sit there and tell me she has no reason to have pain when she has all these new issues in her brain!" I could feel my heart pounding out of my chest.

"Listen, I'm going to schedule you an appointment with Dr. Van Poppel for this upcoming Tuesday, and you can sit and discuss with him your concerns."

Yes, that's going to be perfect, I thought. That way I'll talk face to face with him and get this cleared up. Either way, I was going to make an appointment with Dr. Greenfield up in New York. According to the Chiari Facebook page I was in, he was the closest Chiari expert, the best of the best along with Dr. Grant. I needed his opinion, and New York was only a two-hour plane ride from us. It was easier than going all the way out to California to see Dr. Grant.

Did Dr. Van Poppel not say anything about the basilar invagination because it was too risky to fix? Or maybe it couldn't even be fixed? Or maybe it wasn't that severe? The first decompression surgery he took out too little bone. She was still vomiting and having apnea, then she had papilledema. So, then he went in and took out more bone and did the duraplasty. She still had papilledema two months later, so he inserted the VP shunt, and we were good for a few months. So, the guy acted ... now, did it work? Well, she hasn't vomited. She doesn't need oxygen at night anymore and she is eating orally. The issues were the headaches and irritability which were preferable over the vomiting, apnea, and aspiration pneumonia. She would have been dead already had he not done all this. Her anatomy is bizarre. I definitely need to go to New York, I thought. I need to get as many opinions as I can. Maybe her brain needed a fresh pair of eyes?

The following morning, I called Dr. Greenfield's office at Weill Cornell in New York City. I explained the situation to them, and they agreed to take a look at Alessia's case. I prepared the package of MRI CDs, operative notes, and medical history and sent it overnight to Dr. Greenfield. His office said they would get back to me within the next couple of days to schedule an appointment.

Meanwhile, I prepared for my appointment with Dr. Van Poppel. I made sure I had all my questions written down and tried to put my frustration aside to be able to hear his thoughts without judgment. I could not just go in there and ask him why he hadn't told me about her basilar invagination. I wanted to ask him what he thought of what I had seen on the images.

I printed out all her MRI reports all the way back to October 2016. I also printed out images showing how her cerebellum had slumped down after the decompressions. I went into Tuesday's appointment, confident that I knew more of the brain than your average mom.

"Hey, little monkey!" he greeted Alessia when he walked into the room. He had seen how hyperactive Alessia was, so he always used to call her a little monkey. He was goofy sometimes. I liked that about him.

"Hi, Dr. Van Poppel!" I said. "I wanted to come back to talk to you about a couple of questions I have." He nodded, and I laid out my paperwork on the table. "The whole reason we agreed to a Chiari protocol MRI was because I thought that some of her behaviors were caused by head pain. We did the MRI and you didn't find anything that would explain head pain. However, I looked back at the images and read the reports, and here it says, 'basilar invagination.'" I pointed to the highlighted word on the report. "Do you see how her brainstem is not straight and has like either a ligament or a bone protruding in it? I wanted to know if you think this could be causing her the head pain that she has, because everything that I read in medical articles states that basilar invagination can be very painful."

I thought he would immediately say something. To my surprise, he kept looking back and forth at the reports and the scans on the computer. He kept scratching his beard and furrowing his eyebrows as he looked at the scans on the computer. "Man, oh man," I heard him whisper. He was speechless. He had no idea what to say. Silence. I was getting nervous as I waited for him to speak.

Did he not look at the scans previously? Why was he so quiet? He was so unreadable. I didn't know what he was thinking. Was he thinking that I was a lunatic and had no idea what I was talking about? Probably. I probably would have thought the same if I were him. I mean, I thought basilar invagination was causing her pain because that's what Deanna had suggested. But I was no neurosurgeon and there was a lot I didn't understand.

"I think she is going to need an occipital cranio-cervical spinal fusion at some point." Wait. What? "I would like to get a CT scan of her skull first, but I do think she is eventually going to need a fusion."

What the fuck? Why didn't he tell me this last week when we met? When he said everything was fine? Was I being too insistent?

"Basilar invagination is not a complication of Chiari, I just think the way this ligament is pushing up on her pons is making its way to cranial cervical instability, so I want to address it before it becomes cranial cervical instability. I think this is just how her bone grew over time due to all the deformities she has." He pressed his lips together.

*Well, shit.*

"Do you think this could be contributing to her behaviors?" I asked as I raised my eyebrows.

"It certainly can. Let's get this CT scan and go from there." He exited the room.

I shook my head in disbelief. We had to get to New York as soon as possible. I needed another opinion from a fresh pair of eyes. Alessia's brain was so complex that I needed more than one opinion.

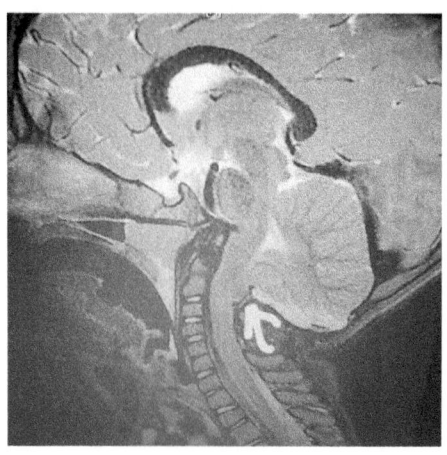
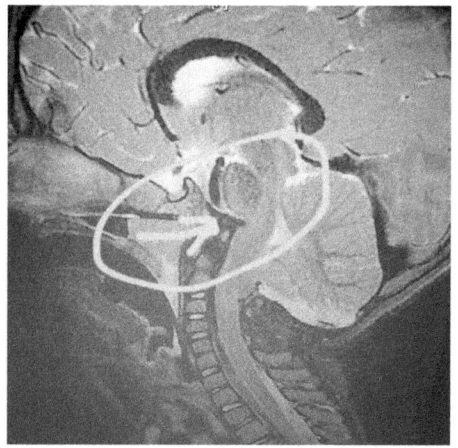

*Alessia's brainstem MRI Images, 2018*
*Photo Credit: Levine Children's Hospital Pediatric Imaging*

## 19

September 28, 2018, was our appointment with Dr. Greenfield at Weill Cornell in New York City. I wasn't 100 percent sure if I wanted to go through the cervical fusion surgery that Dr. Van Poppel had recommended. If Dr. Greenfield agreed that fusion was the way to go, then I would feel more confident with this surgery. There was one piece of advice that I held on to that was given to me by another mother of a medically complex child:

"When you have a child with such a rare diagnosis, you must seek out as many medical opinions as you can. Don't just stay with what the first doctor tells you. You will hear conflicting opinions, but the more opinions you get, the better. Looking at it in different angles will help you make the best decision possible for your child."

By the end of August, we had everything planned and scheduled for our appointment. We would fly to NYC the day before the appointment and come back the day after. We had everything set to stay at the Ronald McDonald House in Manhattan. Everything was good to go. I could not wait to hear Dr. Greenfield's opinion on Alessia's case.

But then Alessia got sick.

Diarrhea. A horrendous case. She would go more than fifteen times a day. Yellow. Liquid, like water. She wasn't potty trained at the time so

I would go through twenty diapers a day. Her bottom was raw. She was in pain. After the fourth day of severe diarrhea, I called Dr. Pineiro, Alessia's GI doctor.

"It's probably just a virus. She has a G tube, so just make sure you give her lots of liquids, Pedialyte, water. Try and do the BRAT diet . . . banana, rice, applesauce, and toast," Dr. Pineiro's physician's assistant said over the phone.

"Yeah, most likely just a virus, hopefully it will clear up soon. Thanks." I hung up the phone and glanced at Alessia, who had a leak from her dirty diaper.

A week later, Alessia still had severe diarrhea. She had lost so much weight. She was pale. I was tired of changing her diaper twenty-five times a day and watching her suffer. We needed to get a stool sample to see what was causing her severe diarrhea. While we waited for the results to come back, Alessia was now running fevers. I was worried. Our appointment with Dr. Greenfield was the following week and Alessia was still ill.

"Adenovirus 40/41," Dr. Pineiro's physician assistant called me with the results after the fiftieth time I had called to inquire on the results. "It's a virus that usually just affects school-aged children, but it can definitely cause severe diarrhea lasting more than ten days. We just have to let the virus run its course."

I could feel my face getting hot as my heart started beater faster.

"It has already been more than ten days," I said as I started pacing from one side of my house to the other. "Isn't there any antibiotic we can give her?" I asked. I was growing inpatient.

"Unfortunately, no. The virus has to run its course. The antibiotics will not do anything to the virus, just keep doing what you're doing. Maybe add a probiotic twice a day."

The diarrhea continued. It wasn't getting any better. By Tuesday, she was paler than I had ever seen her, lethargic, still running fevers. My worry intensified as each day passed. We couldn't go to New York like this.

I took her back to the pediatrician to see if they could run labs on her. She could barely keep her eyes open. We saw another pediatrician because Dr. Squires was out that day. While we were waiting for the lab results, Alessia started vomiting. I remembered the shunt malfunction symptoms. Vomiting and lethargy were two of them. After what seemed like two hours of waiting, the pediatrician came in with the lab results.

"Hey, listen . . . I'm really sorry to say this, but I think you need to take her to the emergency room at Levine's," she said, frowning. "Her white blood count is extremely low. Lower than what I would expect for a child fighting a virus."

*No. Please don't let this be happening.* My heart started pounding. I wiped the sweat that was dripping from my forehead. My stomach started feeling queasy. "Are you serious?" I asked. "Do I have time to go home and drop Sophia off? I don't understand what's going on."

"I really don't know, but I do think she needs a full workup. Levine's emergency room is where she needs to be right now. You have time to go to your house and drop Sophia off. Here's my cell phone number. I will call Levine's ER and give them a heads up that you're coming," she said as she handed me her card.

"Mommy, I don't feel good," Sophia said as she grabbed her tummy. "I think I need to poop."

*Shit.*

"Okay, thank you. I'll head to the hospital as soon as I drop Sophia off." I headed out the door and went straight to the bathroom with Sophia and Alessia. As soon as Sophia sat on the toilet, diarrhea started streaming down. As I wiped her bottom, I heard Alessia exploding her diaper with diarrhea. Or so I thought.

I quickly changed her diaper but saw that her stool had gotten harder. Thank God. I couldn't handle two three-year-olds with severe diarrhea.

I quickly got into the car and called Ronaldo while I drove back home. I was already crying when he picked up. "They want me to take her to the ER. I'm with both girls. I need you to come home and stay with Sophia because I can't take Sophia to the ER. She has diarrhea and she's not feeling good." My voice trembled as I tried to hold back the tears. I was tired. I was exhausted. It had been back-to-back issues with Alessia.

Shit. Traffic!

The cars were at a complete stop. I glanced at the clock. It was right at 5 p.m. Afternoon traffic. Damn it. It was going to take me forever to get to the ER.

"Actually, baby," I said, "let's meet at Levine's ER and you can pick up Sophia there."

"I'm on the other side of town." he said. "It will take me at least forty-five minutes to get to uptown."

I rolled my eyes in frustration.

"Well, just get there whenever you can. I'll wait for you there." Damn it. We were leaving for New York in two days. I needed to call Dr. Greenfield's office and cancel the appointment. There was no way we were going to be getting out of this in time.

## 20

Dr. Greenfield's office was very understanding. They changed our appointment to the following week, which was October 5. Surely, we would be out of the hospital by then and Alessia would be much better, I hoped.

At the ER, they ran all kinds of tests on Alessia. They poked her for blood work. They catheterized her for urine tests . . . There were CT scans . . . an MRI. They did a whole work-up on her. The good thing was she hadn't vomited again, and her diarrhea seemed to be improving, but she was still lethargic, weak, and pale.

"Viral suppression is what we suspect," the ER doctor said as he walked in the room with all the results in his hands. "Her shunt is perfectly fine, her ventricles are within normal limits . . . the only thing concerning is her low white blood count, but we are thinking that it is probably an immune response to the virus that she has been fighting these past couple weeks. She has been fighting against this Adenovirus for so many days that it is likely her immune system has collapsed. We are going to start antibiotics through her IV, as well as fluids. Hopefully, she will make a turn for the better by tomorrow morning."

I bit my lip as I nodded. "How many days will we be here?" I asked. I was thinking about Sophia and her severe diarrhea.

"Well, I'm hoping with antibiotics and IV fluids for the next twenty-four to forty-eight hours, she will improve. If that's the case, I don't see you staying here any longer than Friday." He smiled and walked out of the room.

Thank goodness. Two days was manageable.

I hated the hospital. I hated that Alessia had to stay here. My poor Sophia, not feeling good, and I wasn't even there to comfort her.

Ronaldo and I took turns in the hospital, switching every four to five hours, so I wasn't entirely absent for Sophia and Thiago. Friday came faster than I expected, and thank goodness, Alessia was back to her usual self. Her white blood count was back to normal. Her diarrhea had ceased, and she hadn't vomited again. Thankfully, we were discharged that Friday.

Now I had a week to prepare for our appointment in New York. Thiago and Sophia were going to stay at my mom's house. We were leaving Thursday afternoon to be there Thursday night and go to our appointment Friday morning. I had already gotten letters from her neurosurgeon and her GI doctor, so we wouldn't have any problems with bringing her medical supplies on the plane.

Nothing can go wrong, I thought as I chewed on my nails. Although the thought of taking Alessia on a plane to a different city scared the hell out of me.

"Oh my God. Chill out. It's not like we're going to another country!" Ronaldo whispered to me while we lay in bed. "If anything happens to Alessia while we're there, I'm sure there are hospitals in New York." He wrapped his hands around me.

Alessia fell asleep as soon as the plane took off. She slept the whole flight and didn't wake up until we got to the Ronald McDonald House Thursday night. It was incredible how she could sleep with all the noise of New York

City. I guess there are some perks of being hearing-impaired.

With that long nap also came a period of sleeplessness that lasted till 3 a.m. that night. We had to be at Weill Cornell at 8 a.m. the following morning. That night we only slept for four hours.

Dr. Greenfield is a charming man. He was incredibly knowledgeable and thorough at explaining things. We spent the better part of an hour going over all of Alessia's imaging sequentially and discussing her signs and symptoms at each stage. It appeared to him that she was actually in an upward trajectory. He explained to us that the fact that she had been weaned off of supplemental oxygen and passed a swallow study after her decompression surgeries was a good indication that these interventions had been successful.

"Looking objectively at the MRI scan, there are still residual signs of brainstem compression on the axial cuts, and some apparent degree of cerebellar slumping." Dr. Greenfield pointed to her cerebellum on the image displayed. "I suspect this is all being compounded by the abnormal rotation of her cerebellum low torcula and flat posterior fossa. All very difficult to correct."

*Very difficult to correct . . . No.*

I furrowed my eyebrows.

"I really do think that you need to think strongly about what the rationale for another surgery would be. Further decompression of the brainstem could technically be achieved by tonsillar resection and further reconfiguration of the posterior fossa with a small cranioplasty and muscle flap advancement by plastic surgery. But I honestly don't think fusion surgery is the way to go. The complication rate of a fusion surgery in a child this young . . . is like 100 percent."

I nodded. I thought I was going to throw up.

"I think you need to have more than one conversation and several discussions to really sort out pros and cons of each option. I'd be more than happy to discuss things on the phone with Dr. Van Poppel. I really do think that you need someone local in North Carolina, because I do believe this is certainly going to be a lifelong issue which you will have to periodically address."

This was certainly not what I expected to hear, but I appreciated his honesty and transparency. "So, what can we do about her constant headaches?" I asked. My voice was trembling.

"We could trial a cervical collar for a few months to see if that helps," he replied. "I can order a collar for you to pick up in Charlotte and let's give it a try to see if her headaches subside."

I nodded. I guess we could try that. We didn't have many other options at that point.

I left the appointment more confused than ever. I had been hoping that Dr. Greenfield would have recommended fusion surgery as well. It would have made the decision to have the surgery with Dr. Van Poppel easier. How could two neurosurgeons have such conflicting opinions? One was all for fusion, and the other was against it. Who do I go with?

"Let's enjoy the rest of the day here in NYC. Let's go explore. We can talk about it when we get home." Ronaldo gave me a reassuring hug outside of the clinic. I nodded. He was right. We would have time to discuss things at home. Right now, we should take advantage of the day and go explore. Ronaldo had never been to New York. I had gone twice before and always loved it. I was a city girl and loved the fast-paced lifestyle.

We walked from Weill Cornell all the way to the Twin Towers Memorial. Alessia was in her stroller as we had walked the sixty blocks there. By the time we got to the memorial, we could barely feel our legs from so much walking. It felt like our feet were on fire. Alessia was beyond tired of being in her stroller. The memorial was so peaceful. It was a perfect place to let Alessia out of her stroller to walk around.

There were green areas with benches and trees. Ronaldo and I sat there for a while to rest our legs while Alessia walked around. She was ridiculously cute. She was touching the trees and smiling. I looked over to the "Ground Zero" water fountains where 2,606 people had lost their lives on 9/11. You never know when it's your turn to leave this Earth. We are doing everything possible to keep Alessia alive and these people went to work that day, not even suspecting they would die that day. So much tragedy.

I captured a photo of Alessia leaning on a tree and looking up at the sky. She had the sweetest, most tender smile as she took in the buildings of Manhattan. My eyes filled with tears as I let my thoughts take over:

*I wish you would understand me when I talk to you. I wish I could explain to you what is going on. If only you could talk to me and tell me what you are thinking, what you are feeling. I am so incredibly sorry for all the battles you have had to face in your short life. I am sorry you cannot savor an ice cream cone like a healthy child. I wish we were all in New York on vacation like a normal family, not just the three of us for a doctor appointment that left us more confused than when we got here. I hope you know how much I love you.* A tear ran down my cheek as she looked at me.

The sun was already setting. It was a beautiful sunset in Manhattan. The wind started picking up and it started getting cold. "We should start to head back." I got up from the bench. I could barely feel my legs from all the walking we had done.

"We should probably get an Uber back to the Ronald Mcdonald House," Ronaldo said as he ordered one on his phone.

The water running over my head in the shower felt amazing that night back at the Ronald Mcdonald House. My leg muscles were so sore. I lathered shampoo on my hair and massaged my scalp as I went over all we had discussed with Dr. Greenfield. I had a lot to think about. But I was also incredibly tired.

I lay down on the bed and smelled the clean aroma of the crisp bed sheets. They are so good with cleaning, I thought. I'll make sure to donate to the Ronald McDonald house every time I go to the drive-thru.

I was awakened by Alessia coughing, gagging, and gasping for air. I glanced at the clock: 4 a.m. I felt her forehead. She was burning. Shit. She had a fever, and I didn't have a thermometer. I quickly undressed her and put a wet, cold rag on her forehead. I had Motrin, so I gave her Motrin along with six ounces of water. She was still restless, though, coughing and coughing. The hours went by as Ronaldo and I took turns holding her and trying to put her back to sleep. There was no change. She was sick and by 7 a.m. she hadn't gone back to sleep. She still had a fever and was still coughing. *I'm glad our flight back to Charlotte is in a few hours. I need to get her home.*

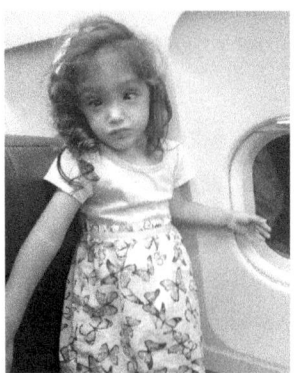

*Alessia on the plane to NY, 2018*

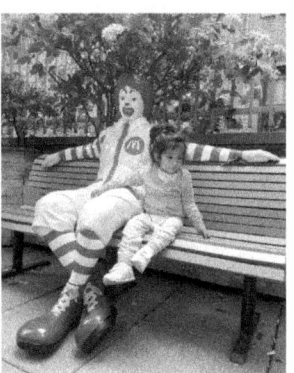

*Ronaldo and Alessia at the Ronald McDonald House NY, 2018 New York Photo Credit: Stephanie Detjen Costabel*

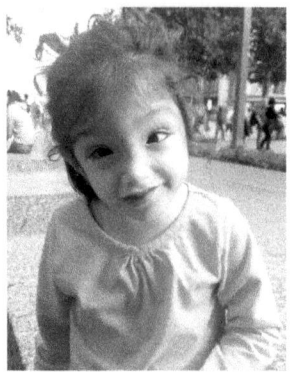

*Alessia in NY, 2018*

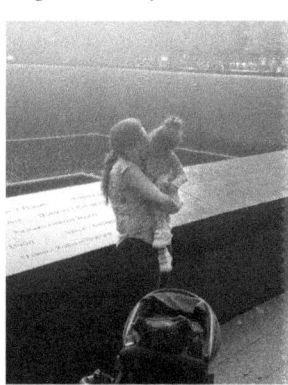

*Alessia and me at the 9/11 Memorial NY, 2018 Photo Credit: Ronaldo Cruz*

## 21

"**D**ouble Pneumonia," Alessia's pulmonologist said. "We will have to start her on a ten-day course of antibiotics and albuterol every four hours. She probably picked up some virus at the airport or in the city."

I nodded. "Most likely the change of weather, perhaps? I don't know. I'm just so glad we're back in Charlotte." I couldn't believe she was sick again. Antibiotics always caused her severe diarrhea. I had already dealt with it for over a month last month. My poor Alessia, she can never catch a break.

After ten days of antibiotics, albuterol, and some more diarrhea, Alessia's pneumonia improved, and she was back to her normal self. Thanksgiving was around the corner. Festivals, pumpkin patches, trees turning orange and red. Fall was in the air.

The eye poking began to become an issue again. I wasn't entirely sure if it was headaches or visual stimulation or sensory seeking, but eventually she managed to develop another corneal ulcer. This time in her right eye.

"It's been a few months," Dr. Daugherty smiled as he walked into the exam room.

"Yes, I know," I said. "I was hoping we didn't have to see you again."

Dr. D laughed.

"We went to New York and got another opinion on Alessia's Chiari. We haven't had any eye issues since last time she had her shunt revision in March." I prepped Alessia on my lap for her eye exam.

He looked in her right eye. "Wow, that's another significant ulcer, Stephanie." He furrowed his brow. "Maybe we should go ahead and check her optic nerves. Did you dilate her eyes before coming?" he asked.

"I sure did," I replied. *God, please don't let her have papilledema.*

Silence fell as he observed her optic nerves. I knew that silence. It usually happened when Dr. D found papilledema. The eye exam usually took a bit longer just to make sure that his findings were accurate.

"I'm sorry, Stephanie," he frowned. "You're going to have to call Dr. Van Poppel. She has swollen optic nerves in both eyes. Her ICP must be high."

*No, not again! I can't believe this is happening again.*

On November 15, 2018, Alessia went in for her sixth brain surgery. Her shunt valve was clogged again with scar tissue, so they had to replace the whole valve.

This was her second shunt revision in one year. Was this really how her life was going to be? Surgery after surgery every year? I felt like I had no more tears left to cry. For a shunt to only last one year was pathetic, but according to the Hydrocephalus Association, shunt failure was common. Unfortunately, there haven't been better treatment options invented for children who have hydrocephalus. Pretty ironic, considering there had been so many medical advancements for plastic surgery. A better treatment than a shunt for something as life-threatening as hydrocephalus hasn't been invented yet. I started getting involved in the Hydrocephalus Association walks to raise money for research for a cure, or at least something more reliable than a shunt. Alessia was added to the hydrocephalus census, and I met some amazing parents of children with hydrocephalus.

It was incredible how much I learned from the hydrocephalus community:

# An Amazing Little Girl with Rhombencephalosynapsis

Approximately 1 million people have hydrocephalus in the US.

There are believed to be 180 different causes.

There is no cure and very little research being done on it. The NIH (National Institutes of Health) spends sixty cents per person with hydrocephalus per year, compared to three hundred dollars per person per year with juvenile diabetes, though the prevalence of each is the same.

The standard treatment, a shunt, was developed in 1956 and has a 50 percent failure rate after just two years, which is the reason so many have to have multiple brain surgeries just to stay alive.

Sixty percent of children with hydrocephalus are not independent as adults and require assistance.

Fifty percent of children with hydrocephalus score 80 or below on standardized intelligence tests.

It costs the United States $1 billion per year in health care costs to treat hydrocephalus.


It finally hit me that this was going to be a lifelong battle. Of course, Alessia not only had hydrocephalus, but she also had Chiari, basilar invagination, Rhombencephalosynapsis, and multiple other disabilities that affected her cranial nerves. I still had no idea what we were going to do about the fusion surgery when Dr. Van Poppel and Dr. Greenfield's opinions were completely contradictory.

"Maybe you should send her scans to Dr. Grant in California," Deanna messaged me. "Maybe he can be the tiebreaker?"

"Yes. Actually . . . that is a good idea. I'm going to call his office," I messaged back. He will be the tiebreaker. If he agrees with Dr. Van Poppel, then I will decide on fusion. If he agrees with Dr. Greenfield, then I will hold off.

I was getting everything ready to send over to Dr. Grant for the second time, when I received a phone call that would change my life.

"Hi, can I please speak to the parents of Alessia Cruz?" A woman's soft voice was on the other end of the line.

"This is Stephanie, Alessia's mom. How can I help you?" I asked.

"This is Mika, from Quality Health Services. You applied for the CAP/C program a couple of months ago and called me to see if I would take Alessia's case."

"Oh yes, I remember now! It's been like three months since I applied. I am assuming we got approved?" I asked.

"You sure did!" she replied. I broke out into a huge grin.

The Community Alternatives Program for Children (CAP/C) provides home and community-based services to children at risk for institutionalization in a nursing home. They provide a pediatric nurse aide as well as respite care, so that the parents of medically fragile kids can take a break. I had applied back when Alessia had the Adenovirus and when my days revolved around her terrible case of diarrhea.

Mika would become one of my best friends and my right hand, my go-to person, my emotional and psychological support. She would make my life more manageable and advocate tirelessly for Alessia. She would be the only other person in the world, besides me, that would know every single medical detail and needs of Alessia. She would help me problem-solve and brainstorm on ways to improve Alessia's quality of life. She would end up lifting a heavy weight off my shoulders. Mika has been the greatest asset to Alessia's team.

The following week, Mika came to our house to meet us and to complete the intake paperwork. She was young, beautiful, and full of energy. She looked at Alessia with a glow in her eyes so I could see how she genuinely cared. She had a strong vocation to help others. I knew from the first day I met her that she was going to be special, and we would have a lifelong friendship. We spent three hours going over all of

Alessia's multiple medical diagnoses and history. She was interested in learning about each illness and took her time asking questions to better understand Alessia's needs.

"I think you should be approved for twenty hours of pediatric nurse care per week, and 720 hours of respite per year," she said. She pointed to where I needed to sign. "That will give you a good break for you to take care of yourself."

I took a deep breath for what felt like the first time in years.

Alessia was not a child who was wheelchair-bound—she was very mobile, extremely strong-willed, and curious. The nurse the nursing agency would match her with had to be someone who had the energy to run around after Alessia and wouldn't mind being outside. Alessia spent 80 percent of her day outside—she loved being outside. She played tag with the trees. She rode her scooter outside. She jumped on the trampoline constantly. Unfortunately, she had absolutely no danger awareness. She would go out in the middle of the street to ride her scooter. One day, I left the front door unlocked and she managed to open the front door and left with her scooter. Five minutes later, I realized the front door was opened and I ran outside. Alessia was already two blocks away in the middle of the street! It was a very scary five minutes. The desperation ran through my veins that day; after that incident we put bolt locks on all the doors.

Alessia was wild and ridiculously stubborn. It was her way or no way. She didn't like wearing shoes and would take them off, no matter how many times you would put them on. She never left her glasses on, even though she had to use them to help with the coordination of her eyes. It's called Strabismus. Her left eye would always turn inward towards her nose. Strabismus was a common symptom of RES. Glasses were supposed to help get her eyes to track better and hopefully uncross themselves.

She loved pulling the leaves off my plants, and no matter how many times we would say "No," she didn't care. She would do whatever she wanted to do, whenever she wanted to do it. I credit her strong personality and resilience to what helped her bloom. She didn't let anything stop her and was fiercely independent.

Alessia could not be left alone, not even for five minutes. She would climb on the countertops and try to reach the toaster oven or a silver knife or a spoon, anything shiny that caught her attention. She loved water. You couldn't leave a glass of water anywhere because she would find it and throw it to the floor to see the glass break and the water splashing all over. She was amused by it. I could never figure out why. I wasn't sure if it was auditory stimulation to hear the glass breaking on the floor, or the adrenaline of seeing the water splash. We had to be extra careful with her. She was ridiculously smart and incredibly fearless.

Out of all the nurses I met with, there was one that caught my attention. She was relatively quiet, but I noticed that she interacted a lot more with Alessia then the other nurses had when they came for the interviews. Her name was Bee and she had been a medical assistant at a hospital. She was able to do the hours that I wanted: 9 a.m. to 1 p.m. Monday through Friday. I figured she could go for a walk with Alessia in the mornings and watch her while I went and did grocery shopping and cleaned the house. I wanted Bee to do some sign language with Alessia. Maybe Alessia would learn some signs now that she had someone consistently teaching them to her.

At first Alessia seem to like her a lot, and everything was going well, but eventually Bee started showing up late every day. Some days she wouldn't even show up. She started to be unreliable, so after about a month I had to let her go. I later found out that she wasn't even a CNA, which was what CAP/C required to provide a paid aide.

"You know, we could always do the 'Consumer Direction' program," Mika said when I called her to tell her about Bee not being a good fit.

## An Amazing Little Girl with Rhombencephalosynapsis

"Consumer Direction is a program where you can hire whoever you want to hire, and you don't have to go through a nursing agency."

"Don't they have to have a CNA or an RN degree?" I asked.

"Not when you are in the Consumer Direction program. You just have to find the person. The only requirement through the Consumer Lite program is they have to be CPR certified. You do the interview. You do the timesheets, and then an outside provider does the pay stubs. If it is something that you want to try, I can set you up for the program," she said.

I thought about it for a moment. "Well, I do know a lot of people on Facebook. Maybe if I post it somebody will apply?" I put the phone on speaker as I scrolled through my Facebook friends. "Or at least share the post, you know?"

"I mean, I think it's worth a try after what happened with Bee. Some of my clients have a family member that they pay to be the aide. If somebody is looking for a job and it's a family member, you will trust them more," Mika said. She was so good at advising me.

Mika enrolled me in the Consumer Direction program and after a few weeks I was ready to start searching for an aide. "Alessia is hiring," I posted on my personal Facebook page. "Please Share: Twenty hours per week, schedule is flexible. $16 dollars per hour. Must be physically active and full of energy. Alessia likes to ride her scooter around the block and loves to be outside. Must be okay with that. Must be willing to help with her G tube feedings, as well as some play therapy using sign language. I will train you. If you're interested in this rewarding experience of helping a special needs child, please PM me." I attached the cutest picture of Alessia. Who could resist her beautiful face?

After about two days I had some people that were interested. One of them was a woman who had worked with Ronaldo. Her name was Diane, and Ronaldo spoke very highly of her. She was currently studying nursing at UNC Charlotte and was interested in working with Alessia. I interviewed her and immediately liked her. She was full of energy and interested in working with Alessia. She also knew some sign language, and the fact she was studying nursing was a huge plus. I didn't think twice and called her the next day to offer her the job.

Diane was reliable, never late, hardly took any breaks, and was eager to learn. She tried constantly to play with Alessia and teach her sign language. Alessia was hard to get to interact, but in her own way she showed she was content with Diane. I showed Diane how to tube feed Alessia. She was doing great, and I was happy. Diane, on the other hand, was a little worried. She felt she wasn't doing much and couldn't quite handle that Alessia was so inattentive and stubborn in her own ways.

It came to me as an utter surprise when Diane quit two weeks into the job.

I had no idea she wasn't happy being Alessia's aide. In those two weeks I had learned to trust her. Alessia learned to love her as well.

"I really hate to do this," she texted me the night before she was scheduled to come. "I have grown to love Alessia, but I just don't think I am qualified enough to do the work that is required. I am sorry."

I swallowed hard as I read her text. I didn't have the energy to reply. She evidently did not want to work for us anymore, so I wasn't going to push it, even though I thought her reasoning was silly—she'd been doing a great job. "Okay thanks for letting me know," I replied and shut my phone off.

"Why?" Mika asked over the phone. "What is so difficult about taking care of Alessia? I mean, you put on the post that they have to be physically active and that she has special needs, so obviously she wasn't going to be an attentive, normal three-year-old child."

"I don't know," I replied. "I hadn't really asked her to do anything except watch her and use some signs whenever she played with her, that's it. I don't know why she got discouraged."

"Isn't there a family member that might help you out?" Mika asked.

"I could ask my mom, but she has a full-time job already. She'd only be able to come help me a couple hours over the weekend. I guess we could do that for now until I find someone who has more availability during the week." I thought about what my mother would say when I asked her.

"I wish we were in Colorado and CAP/C could just pay me to be her caregiver. I would use that money to pay someone to come and clean the house or make us food. That would be a tremendous help." I remember reading an article about Colorado paying the parents of special-needs children as their caregivers. In North Carolina, special-needs children in the CAP/C program must be eighteen years old to hire their parents to be their caregivers. Before that age it was not allowed.

"That's true, but unfortunately here in North Carolina you can't do that. Actually, there is an advocacy group of parents of special-needs children that are trying to change the law here, but they haven't had much success in the last couple of years. It's ridiculously hard to find a nurse that will be a good fit."

Mika helped me make decisions, and we decided to put my mother on as an aide so as not to lose the hours that had already been approved by Medicaid. It was going to be temporary, though, until I could find someone that would be able to come during the week.

Most of 2019 was quiet. Alessia only had one procedure in April that was to remove her adenoids and tonsils—a sleep study revealed she had severe obstructive apnea. Alessia's Ear, Nose, and Throat doctor that did the procedure was surprised to find that Alessia was missing a tonsil;

she only had her right tonsil. The left tonsil apparently never developed. Even after removing her adenoids and the only tonsil she had, she still required a CPAP machine to sleep. The muscles in her airway were just too weak and floppy and the obstruction was too significant for her to discontinue CPAP therapy.

We had a couple of other discussions with Dr. Van Poppel about fusion surgery, but I decided to wait until she was older. We consulted with two other neurosurgeons, one at Duke and the other at UNC Chapel Hill. Both had conflicting opinions about fusion surgery at Alessia's age. Dr. Grant from California reached out to me after I had sent all of her scans and he agreed with Dr. Greenfield that fusion wasn't the way to go for now, so we decided to just monitor with yearly scans until she was older, or her basilar invagination progressed.

We applied for a wish from the Make-A-Wish Foundation. I thought a hydrotherapy hot tub would be the wish Alessia would ask for if she could speak. Her love for water was incredible. It would take a couple of months to get our wish, but I was in no rush. Alessia was doing well. She was going to start school in August. There was an Exceptional Children's Program at an elementary school nearby. Alessia had started Equine Therapy and she loved it. She loved horses. Those animals were therapy to her soul.

We had a lot of good things coming up that fall. I decided we were all in need of a vacation. We had many things to celebrate: Thiago was turning eight on August 17, Alessia had been illness free and out of the hospital for more than six months, and my mother's birthday was on August 16. Why not? I thought. Sophia and Thiago had never been on a plane. We hadn't been on an actual vacation for years. "I love the idea!" Ronaldo hugged me and kissed my temple when I told him my plan, and he smiled from ear to ear. So, on August 15, 2019, Ronaldo, my mother, my stepdad, Thiago, Sophia, Alessia, and I boarded a plane to Puerto Rico.

# An Amazing Little Girl with Rhombencephalosynapsis

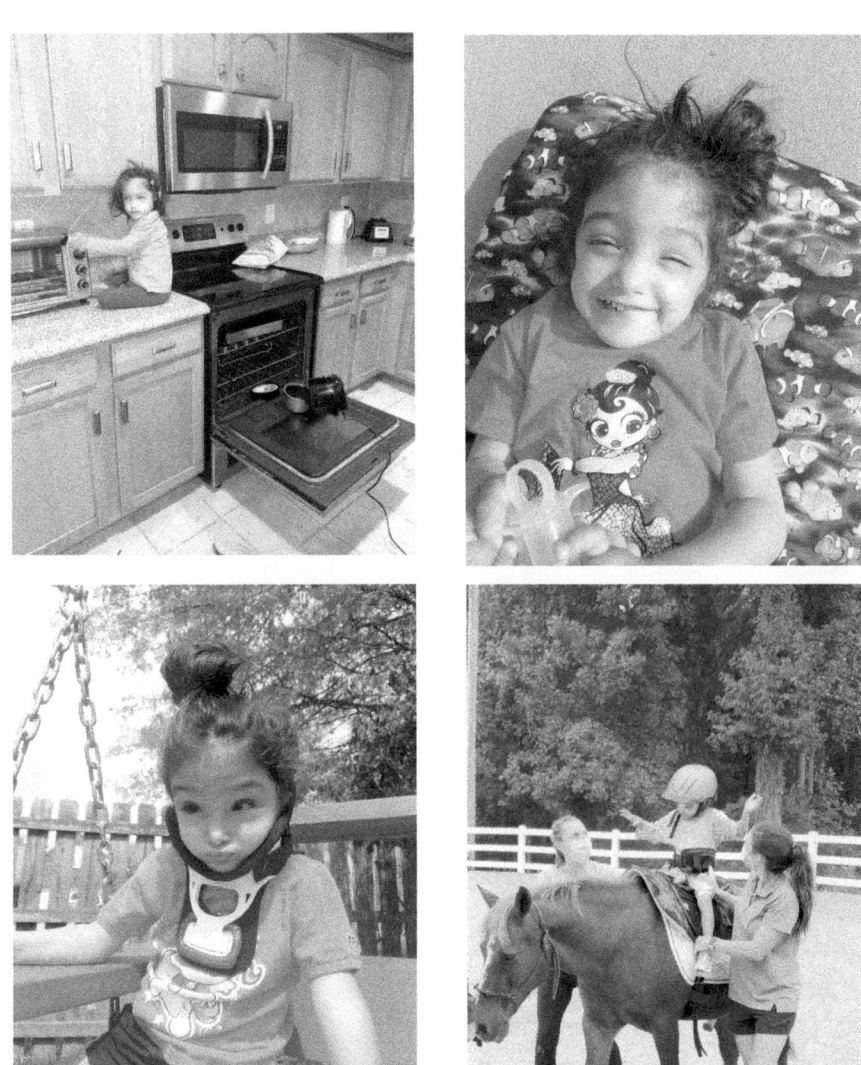

*2018. All Photo Credits: Stephanie Detjen Costabel*

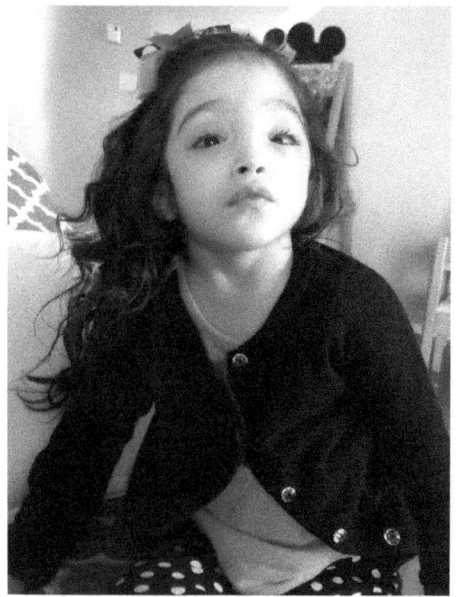
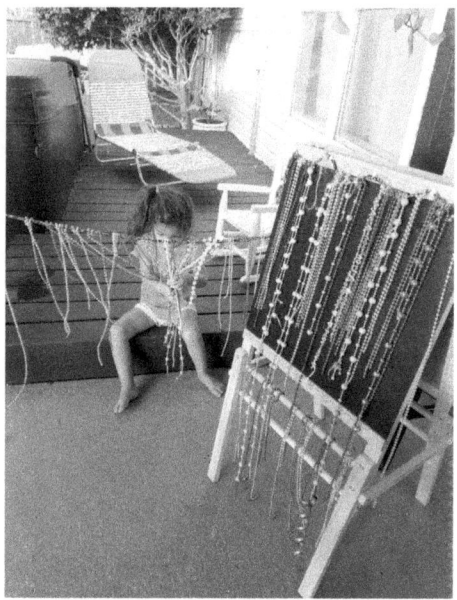

*Alessia waiting for her shunt revision, 2018*

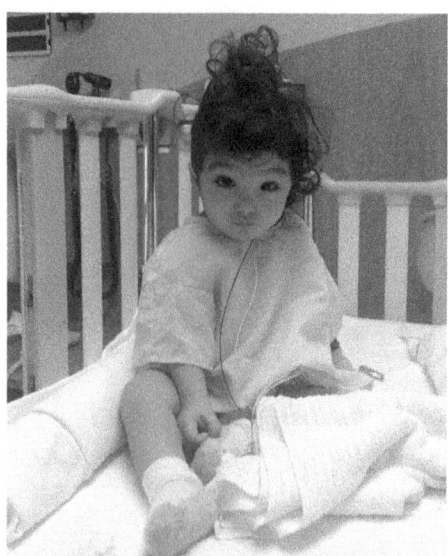
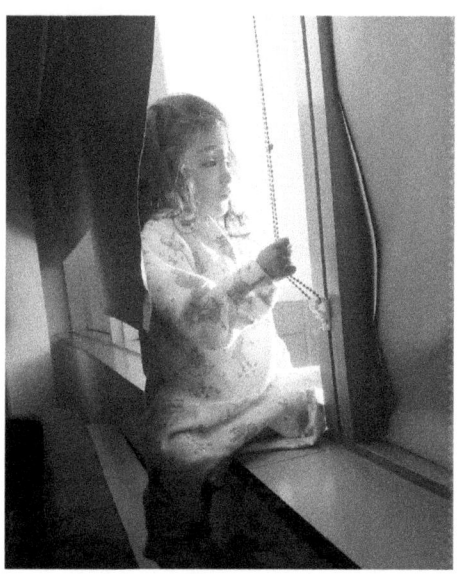

*Alessia after her shunt revision, 2018*

*Alessia looking out the window at Levine after her shunt revision, 2018*

*All Photo Credits: Stephanie Detjen Costabel*

## 22

We rented a beautiful house in Puerto Rico with a large balcony overlooking the sea. It had a comfortable hammock that Alessia loved to swing in. The house was rustic and incredibly cozy. The warm tropical breeze in Puerto Rico was therapy for the soul. I had never seen my children so happy. The water of the beaches was clear and turquoise, more vivid than anything I'd ever seen. The sand was white, like sugar. You could walk in the ocean for miles and still be in shallow water on the beach we went to. Alessia was like a fish, wanting to be in the water constantly. She laughed, smiled, and even tried to swim. Seeing her so happy and enjoying life brought so much joy to my heart. Spending quality time with my mother and stepfather was also rewarding. My mother and stepfather stayed one night with Alessia while Ronaldo, Thiago, Sophia, and I went to downtown San Juan for dinner. We had an incredible night, and although I missed Alessia, I knew I had to balance my time with my other two children. I hadn't had a day alone with them and Ronaldo ever since Alessia was born. My mother did an excellent job keeping Alessia entertained while we were at dinner.

It was the best vacation I ever had with the girls and Thiago. I was sad to leave. There is something about the Caribbean that makes you want to stay forever.

By the end of our vacation, Alessia's corneas were completely white from the salt water. Her eyes did not look good. They weren't clear at all. The need to put her head and eyes underwater gave her immense relief. She would not close her eyes in the ocean or at a pool, or even in the bathtub. We constantly were removing her hands and her fingers from her eyeballs and would even put on arm restraints to prevent her from scratching her corneas. But she always outsmarted us, finding a way to relieve that sensory deficit she had in her eyeballs. If she could not scratch her corneas with her fingers, she would use her toes or drag her eye on the carpet or on the cement. If she were out of the water at the beach, she would put sand in her eyes. Five days in Puerto Rico was sufficient. If we would have stayed there any longer, she would surely have damaged her eyes completely.

Nobody was able to figure out why children with Rhombencephalosynapsis had the need to constantly dig at their eyes. Not the University of Washington, Neurosurgery, Ophthalmology, the Developmental Pediatrician . . . not one person knew the exact reason. Everyone had their suspicions and opinions. RES'ers eye poked because of headaches, boredom, for visual stimulation, for sensory input, eye dryness, visual impairment, constipation, stomachache . . . but science never was able to confirm the exact reason why this behavior was so common in kids with RES.

The fact that she was missing her left trigeminal nerve and was unable to feel her cornea was extremely dangerous and was the cause of her deteriorating vision loss. She had corneal scarring in both eyes. I was extremely worried that Alessia would end up blind.

Alessia started Pre-K at Hickory Grove Elementary School in the Exceptional Children's classroom. It was a bittersweet day, as I had been with her 24/7 for the past four and a half years. Letting her go to school and be in somebody else's care for a school day made shivers run down my spine.

I got Alessia dressed in her school uniform and prepared her feeding tube supplies, my legs shaking with nerves. As always, she had a meltdown when I tried to put her shoes on. I tried five times and five times she removed them. I put her shoes and socks in the book bag and decided I was just going to take her in bare feet. God, Alessia, why do you have to be so stubborn?

While I was getting Alessia ready, Sophia had already brushed her teeth, washed her face, and gotten dressed. She was going to go to the Albemarle Road Weekday School, which was a church Pre-K program from 9:30 a.m. to 1:30 p.m., Monday through Friday. Sophia loved it there and the teachers were amazing. She had no other option except to learn how to be independent. My heart ached. I hope she will one day understand how incredibly thankful I was that she was such an easy child and so independent.

I dropped Sophia off first. She was so excited. "How do I look, Mama?" she asked as she put her long braid over her right shoulder. She was so sassy and girlie.

"Like a princess." I smiled and kissed her cheek. She waved at me as she walked into the front doors of the school. My sweet Sophia. She was getting so big. Her hair was so long and luscious.

My hands shook as I drove to Alessia's school. Please let her have a good first day of school! I was so nervous. Nervous because having a child enter kindergarten with no vocabulary whatsoever was terrifying. She couldn't tell me if she had a good day or a bad day. She couldn't talk about her day. If she was cold, hot, hungry, thirsty, uncomfortable, she could not tell her teacher absolutely anything because she was nonverbal. The thought of that scared the shit out of me.

I carried Alessia into her classroom. She loved to be carried around. She was four years old but still like a toddler. She loved when I held her.

"Hi, Alessia!" Miss Switzer gave us a warm smile. She was so young, beautiful, and full of energy. I immediately warmed up to her.

"Is it okay if I stay a few minutes?" I asked. My eyes were watery. I was about to burst into tears.

"I really would like to say no, but I completely understand. You can stay for a couple of minutes, that's fine," Miss Switzer replied.

To my surprise, Alessia went straight to a swing they had in the room and was as happy as she could be swinging herself. I was in much more pain than she was. She started exploring the room and didn't even look back at me when I waved to her goodbye.

"She will be fine," Miss Switzer said. "Don't worry. She is in good hands."

I swallowed hard, nodded, and left the classroom.

As soon as I got in my car, tears started pouring down my cheeks.

I sat in the parking lot for over an hour. I wanted to be close by just in case anything happened.

"You're being paranoid," Ronaldo said when he called me to see how Alessia was. "Go out and do some grocery shopping or go get your nails done or go back to the house. Nothing is going to happen to her. Geez, relax a little!"

"You're right, I'm going to go home for a little bit and clean," I said as I started the car. He laughed over the phone. "Cleaning is what you always do."

Back at home, the silence in the house was creeping me out. It was the first time in four years that I had been alone in my house. What the hell is wrong with me? I should be enjoying the peace.

I prepared myself a coffee and sat outside, staring at the clouds. It was beautiful outside. August was usually hot, but that morning was pleasant. I was searching for a song to put on YouTube on my phone when a call came in from Hickory Grove Elementary School.

Shit.

"Hello?" I immediately answered the call.

"Hi, Mrs. Costabel?"

"This is her," I replied.

"This is Debbie, the nurse at Hickory Grove Elementary School." My heart started racing. "Alessia fell while she was in physical therapy, and she busted her lip. She is fine. I don't think she needs stitches, but it would probably be a good idea if you came to pick her up."

Suddenly my knees felt like jelly and my stomach felt queasy.

"I'll be there in five minutes." I hung up the phone.

Are you freaking kidding me? This was her first day of school. This wasn't how it was supposed to go. Not even two hours had gone by since I dropped her off. Breathe, Stephanie, I said to myself, before you kill someone at the school.

I stormed into the school office.

Miss Switzer was holding Alessia with an ice pack over her lip. The white polo shirt that I had ironed that morning had bright red blood stains all down the front. The physical therapist was there, as well as the nurse and the principal of the school. They all looked worried. Probably petrified of what I was going to say to them. Alessia, on the other hand, was acting like nothing had happened. She was content in Miss Switzer's arms. She seemed calm and had no tears in her eyes.

It didn't surprise me. Alessia had fallen so many times at the house, but she never cried. It's like she never felt pain. This was common with kids that had RES—their pain tolerance was extremely high.

"We are so, so, extremely sorry." Miss Switzer's voice was trembling. She was so scared I actually felt bad for her.

I swallowed hard before I spoke. "Listen, accidents can happen to anyone. It's okay. She is fine and that is what matters. I do think she needs to have a one-to-one aid, though, with her at all times." I glanced over to the principal. "Alessia is wild and so incredibly stubborn. She will climb on the desks, put herself in danger and not even know it. It is incredibly hard to keep her safe without constantly watching her. She needs a nurse or a CNA constantly watching her. I don't think Miss Switzer and her assistant with eleven other students can guarantee Alessia will stay safe here. Please. She needs an aide here at school to be with her at all times."

"I totally agree with you," the principal said as he looked over to Miss Switzer. "But for her to have an aide there is a process. CMS has to collect what is known as 'data points.' They have to observe her for a certain amount of time and document how many times during the day she needs one-to-one assistance. Now," he cleared his throat, "there is a school called the Metro School that is dedicated to children that have complex needs like Alessia."

"I've heard of the Metro School," I interrupted him. "But I wanted to give her a chance at a normal school. If she has a one-to-one aide, she can prosper in a normal school setting."

"Well, then we should start the application for a nurse and start collecting data points," he said.

I called Mika as soon as I left the school. "What more proof do they need? I mean, she busted her lip open within the first two hours of her first day?"

I was now extremely nervous to send her back to school.

"When is her eye strabismus surgery?" Mika asked.

"Two weeks."

"Let's give them time to gather their data points. She will be out of school for a week due to her surgery and the rest of the days you can just send her half days, from 9 a.m. to 12 p.m. I mean, I am sure they are going to pay more attention to her after today's fall. They are probably scared to death now."

I laughed. Mika was always right and knew how to help me look at the situation in different angles.

Strabismus was common in the RES world. In Alessia's case, it was her left eye that would turn inward. Strabismus affects a child's depth perception. They can also see double, blurry, and have sensitivity to light. All these symptoms can produce headaches. We tried patching her right eye to get the left eye to align better. Her right eye was her good eye. By patching the right eye, the eye muscles of the left eye would get stronger. She would need to use it more to be able to see. We had to patch her good eye eight hours each day, but after a few weeks Alessia grew tired of it and would rip the eye patch off. She had a degree of numbness on her face due to the underdeveloped trigeminal nerve, so it was not painful to her to rip tape off her face.

We decided to go through with the strabismus surgery. It was an outpatient procedure during which they would tighten the muscles of her left eye so her eye alignment would be straighter; that way both eyes would work in coordination with each other to see better.

Unfortunately, with the strabismus surgery came an increase in Alessia's eye poking addiction. By October, she had a significant corneal ulcer in her left eye. We saw Dr. Daugherty every two days to make sure the ulcer was healing. After about three weeks, he referred us to a corneal specialist. Alessia's ulcer had gotten infected, and it was getting deeper. Basically it looked like it was melting her cornea.

"Have you heard of Oxervate?" I asked the corneal specialist, Dr. Viber.

As usual, I had done my own research before the appointment, searching for a cure. I had heard about Oxervate a few months ago: it was a new eye drop that had recently been approved by the FDA to help the healing of problematic ulcers. It contained Cenegermin, a man-made form of a substance made by your body, used to help maintain and make more nerve cells in your eyes. My hope was that it would help Alessia's ulcer heal.

"I can prescribe Oxervate, and we can try it, but I'm not exactly sure if it would work for her. The eye drops are designed for people who were born with sensation in their cornea that have lost it over the years. In her case, she was born without sensation. But I do think it's worth a shot. If you want me to prescribe it I can. What would really help her is a tarsorrhaphy."

"Yes, Dr. D has talked to me about sewing her eyelids together. But I am not going to do that." I crossed my arms.

Had I known a tarsorrhaphy would have saved her vision I wouldn't have thought twice about it. But at the time, I had no idea how bad her corneas were going to get without the tarsorrhaphy. The eye is an amazing organ. Sewing the eyelids partially together would have helped maintain the eye moisture and better protect it from exposure or disease, creating a perfect atmosphere for the cornea to heal.

"Well, I also think it would be a great idea to get her on serum tears," Dr. Viber said.

"What are serum tears?" I asked.

"Serum tears are eye drops made out of a patient's own blood. Serum is the clear fluid that remains after the cells and most of the proteins are removed from the blood. These drops have healing and nurturing properties beyond that of commercially available artificial tears. It's worth a shot if you would like to try it."

I nodded. What did I have to lose?

"Now, you do have to go to a compounded pharmacy in Hickory to get these tears made. They would have to extract blood from her. You will have to pick them up in the afternoon after they are made."

"If it can help heal her ulcer, I don't mind at all."

All these medications were novel. There had been very few children that had actually used them. It was scary. But her eye looked so bad that I was desperate beyond measure to try to preserve her vision.

## An Amazing Little Girl with Rhombencephalosynapsis

One of the doctors at Duke Eye Center had written an article revolving around the use of Oxervate and its success rate in patients with neurotrophic keratoplasty. Dr Victor Perez was an established clinician-scientist investigator in the field of Ocular Immunology and Ocular Surface diseases and was the director of the Foster Center for Ocular Immunology. He was the best of the best when it came to Ocular Immunology. Surely, he would help. I needed to take Alessia to see him. But he was a remarkably busy man. I scheduled an appointment with Dr. Perez, but the soonest was one month out. In the meantime, Alessia's eye kept deteriorating.

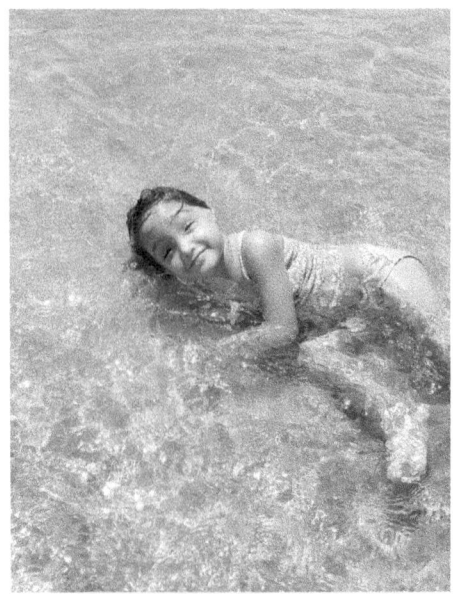

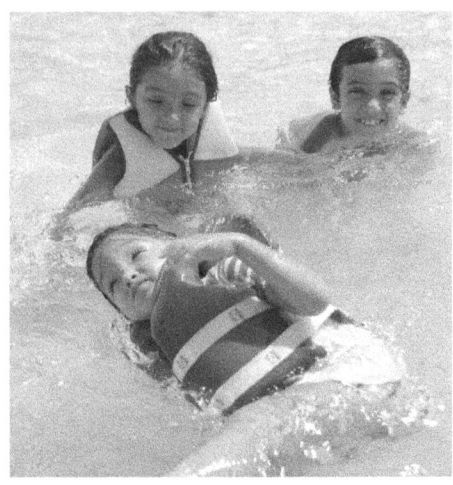

*Puerto Rico, 2019*

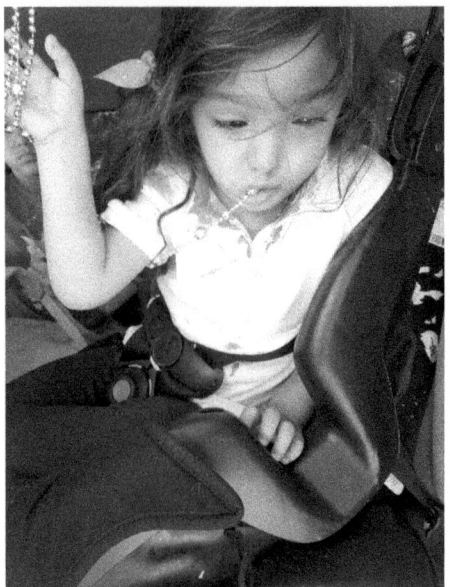

*Alessia's busted lip on her first day of school, 2018*

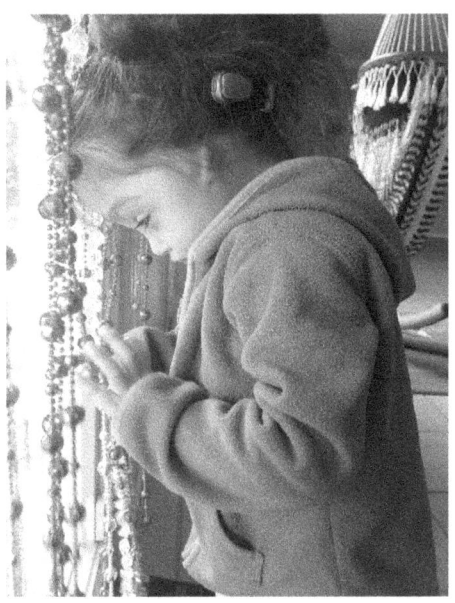

*Alessia playing with her favorite thing in the whole wide world: beads*

*All Photo Credits: Stephanie Detjen Costabel*

## 23

"Yes, I know this is an extremely novel eye drop and it takes longer when it comes to Medicaid to get it approved, but I don't have ten thousand dollars right now to pay for these eye drops, and it's an emergency. My daughter is losing vision in her eye because of a non-healing ulcer . . . please." My hands shook as I tried to hold the phone still. I held back my tears.

It had been two weeks and we still had not received the Oxervate eye drops. We had the serum tears that I was administering six times a day, along with her antibiotic eye drops and steroids. Nothing was working. My days revolved around putting eye drops in her eye every hour. But her corneal ulcer was getting worse, and her cornea kept melting.

Mika made some phone calls to Dompe Pharmaceuticals, the company that provided the Oxervate drops, to see if she could have any luck with them when I didn't. We were waiting for Medicaid to approve payment for them. Mika was insistent. She would fight for her clients. She was incredibly responsible and proactive. Thanks to her persistence, we received the Oxervate drops a week before Alessia's appointment with Dr. Perez.

Between the Oxervate drops, the serum tears, the antibiotic drops, and the steroid drops, I was administering one drop per hour from the moment Alessia woke up to the moment she went to sleep. I was dreaming of eye drops. The alarm on my phone was constantly reminding me she needed an eye drop. My life revolved around putting eye drops in her eye. Her eye was my priority. I knew she was at risk for perforating her eye since her ulcer was so deep. I was exhausted from worrying about it. I had read that when an eye ulcer got so deep it could potentially perforate and deflate. Known as a "globe rupture," you could lose your whole eye if it wasn't treated urgently.

Dr. Perez was charming, smart, educated, and down to earth. He was from Puerto Rico, so we had the Spanish culture/language connection. He was humble and genuine. I liked him from the first day I met him.

"You have to give it time," he told me. "Oxervate is the best thing for her right now. I'm surprised you got the drops so soon." He examined her ulcer. "Oxervate is what is going to help it heal. Give it time. It's going to heal. I want to see her in about two weeks. You said you see your local ophthalmologist next week, right?" he asked.

"Yes, we see Dr. Viber in Charlotte next week."

In North Carolina, the best place for children's eyecare is the Duke Eye Center. The issue was that it was two hours away from Charlotte. So, if we could come for follow-up appointments every other week to Duke, it would certainly help save money in gas and time. My sister lived about forty-five minutes away from Duke in Raleigh, so I had a place to stay if I needed to, but Alessia didn't like sleeping anywhere else other than her bed at home. Her bed was enclosed in a tent-like breathable fabric. She was used to sleeping in her bed and felt secure in it.

After seeing Dr. Perez, my next appointment was with Dr. Viber the following week to check her ulcer. Dr. Viber was extremely knowledgeable, but also so extremely busy. In Charlotte, there are not enough corneal specialists for the population. Dr. Viber was an adult corneal specialist. He could check up on her eye and all, but he wasn't pediatrics.

The best eye care was ultimately at Duke.

"It's deep," Dr. Viber said as he examined her ulcer. "I think you need to go to Duke ASAP. The only thing that I can do is shut her eye completely, a total tarsorrhaphy. It is dangerously close to perforation." Dr. Viber sat on his chair, a deep look of concern on his face.

It was Friday. *How am I supposed to get her in to see someone at Duke over the weekend? He had never said that before about her ulcer: it must be bad.*

Nothing had helped, not the Oxervate, not the antibiotic, not the steroids, not the serum tears. Her eye was perforating, and I had to act before she ended up losing her eye.

Dr. Davis was the resident on call at the Duke Eye Center's emergency line. "Come tomorrow morning and we'll take a look at it. If she needs a corneal transplant to save her eye, we will do it in the morning. Just make sure she doesn't eat anything past midnight. Dr. Perez is out of the country and won't be back until next week. But Dr. Williams is here, and he can do a transplant if she needs it," he said, when I called Duke that same Friday.

I had made plans with the kids that weekend. I was going to take them to the North Carolina Zoo. They were excited to go. My mother was in Spain with my stepfather on vacation. Shit.

I was going to have to take them. My sister would come pick Thiago and Sophia up from Duke in the morning, and I would stay with Ronaldo and Alessia while they figured out what they were going to do.

That Saturday morning you could feel Fall in the air. "It seems like every fall something happens with Alessia. Last year it was the adenovirus and the diarrhea. Now this year it's her eye." I glanced at Ronaldo hoping he would have some words of encouragement.

"Well, let's just get there and see what they say. Maybe they don't need to do surgery." He pressed his lips together and continued driving.

Yeah right, not even he could believe that.

We arrived exactly at 8 a.m. at the Duke Eye Center. Dr. Davis was waiting for us at the front. The clinic was closed. The only people there were Dr. Davis, Ronaldo, Alessia, and me. He led us into one of the pediatric eye exam rooms. "Okay, let's see what's going on." He looked in her eye with his ophthalmologist flashlight. "It doesn't look good," he said. "Let me call Dr. Williams, the corneal specialist on call. I'll be right back." He exited the room.

It was the longest hour of my life. Dr. Williams needed to come and look at her eye and give the okay for the corneal transplant. They also needed to have the anesthesia team ready.

At around 1 p.m., everything was ready to go. Since Alessia was Dr. Perez's patient, Dr. Williams made sure to get his recommendations beforehand.

"Dr. Perez doesn't think Alessia is ready for a full corneal transplant, so what we are going to do is get some tissue from the Eye Bank and fill up the hole. The goal here is to preserve her eye because if it ends up perforating, we will eventually have to remove her eye," Dr. Williams said.

We had no other choice. We had to do the corneal transplant or else she would lose her eye. "Please, God, let everything go well," I whispered as I kissed Alessia's cheek. It was the first time she was having surgery at Duke. I was in unknown territory. I was nervous, scared, sad . . . but we were at the best place we could possibly be at. The ball was in their court now. We could only hope for the best.

I paced back and forth in the waiting room. It was a Saturday. There was nobody there except us. The entire procedure took four hours. I didn't go back to see her until 6:00 p.m. that day.

"I am so glad you guys brought her in today," Dr. Williams said as he arrived in Post-Op Recovery. "Her eye perforated on the OR table. If you guys wouldn't have brought her in, surely she would have lost her eye."

I put my hand on my heart. Thank God she didn't.

"I'd like to see her tomorrow morning to make sure that the corneal transplant is stable. We did a partial temporary tarsorrhaphy to help the transplant heal. It's temporary, I just put two stitches on the outer corner of her eyelids. We can remove them in a couple of weeks. I also added an Amniotic Membrane Transplant to help with healing. It's cells from an amniotic membrane donor. It helps it heal faster." He drew a picture on a sheet of paper showing me every single detail of what they did. I really appreciated how incredibly thorough he was at explaining every single detail to me. Not many doctors take that time. Dr. Williams was amazing. I was impressed by his bedside manner.

We stayed at my sister's house that night to go to the follow-up appointment the following day. I was surprised Alessia was leaving her eye shield on. It seemed like she had relief after the transplant. I wondered if the ulcer had been bothering her all this time because she seemed in great spirits right after her surgery. Unfortunately, because Alessia was under anesthesia the whole afternoon, it made her incredibly hyper during the night, and we did not get any sleep. We drove straight back to Charlotte after the appointment. We had to come back the following Wednesday to see Dr. Perez. When I looked at her eye, I was amazed by the precision of the stitches around her pupil. A pupil I hadn't seen in over a month. The corneal ulcer had so much scar tissue it was hazy and white, making the pupil hard to see. Her cornea looked so much better. I sighed. Thank God we were done with her ulcer. Now we could continue on with our lives. I was so relieved and so incredibly tired at the same time.

It's physically exhausting to have a medically complex child. But somehow, your body gets used to the sleepless nights. We got home and I was Alessia's shadow for the whole day. I didn't want her touching her shield or messing with her recently operated eye. She seemed to be in good spirits for the rest of the afternoon, but by nighttime she wasn't herself. She was in pain. I was on top of her pain meds, but nothing seemed to relieve her. Around 9 p.m., she started having explosive diarrhea. Must be the anesthesia, I thought. A couple of days before her corneal transplant, she'd had bouts of diarrhea here and there, but it was nowhere near as bad as it had been the year before when she had the adenovirus.

I gave her some Pepto Bismol and put her down to sleep.

The next morning, Alessia was still not herself. She was still in pain and had diarrhea. By the afternoon she became lethargic. It was Monday.

I went by myself to the appointment with Dr. Perez. Alessia was extremely lethargic. It helped that she was asleep when he came into the room. He was able to examine her eyes without having to fight her.

"It looks good." Dr. Perez smiled.

"Continue with the antibiotic ointments and steroid drops." He put down his ophthalmoscope.

"Do you know if they checked her optic nerves for papilledema while she was under anesthesia for her transplant?" I asked.

"Yes, they did, and she did not have papilledema," he replied.

Probably just a virus then. "She's just been very lethargic and has had some diarrhea these past couple of days." I placed Alessia on my other arm. My right arm had grown numb from carrying her. She was still asleep.

"Her corneal transplant looks good; she could just be tired still from the anesthesia. It has only been four days since her surgery. Let's see her back in about ten days." He smiled and exited the room.

I had this gut-wrenching feeling that something was not right. My motherly instincts never failed. On my drive home, Alessia kept sleeping. Halfway to Charlotte, she briefly woke up and started throwing up. *No.*

I pulled over on the side of the highway and got her out of her car seat. She was drenched in vomit but fell back asleep as soon as I changed her.

# An Amazing Little Girl with Rhombencephalosynapsis

I called Ronaldo. "Something is wrong with Alessia. She vomited and she has been so lethargic all day."

"It's probably still the anesthesia," he said.

"No, something feels off. If she throws up again, I am going to take her to the ER." I pressed on the gas and was now speeding on the highway. I had to get to Charlotte fast.

It's incredible how my instincts with Alessia have always been right. Our connection has always been miraculous. It was so much stronger than a normal motherly instinct. I knew deep down in my heart that something was not right. What I did not know at the time was just how incredibly ill she was about to get. She was knocking on death's door and the worst day of my life was about to unravel before my eyes.

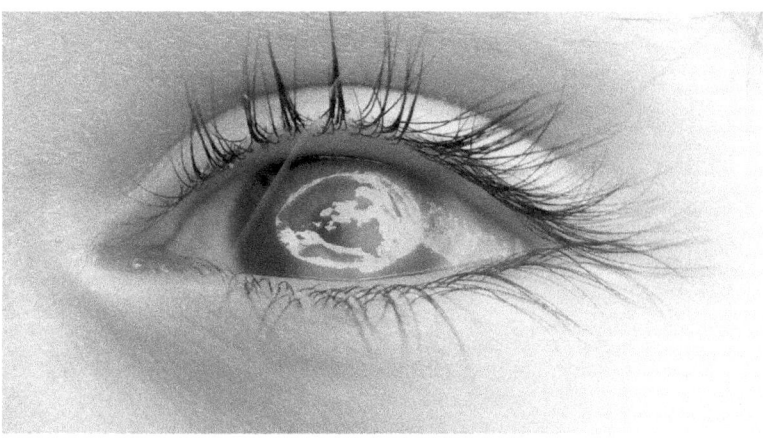

*Alessia's perforated eye. Photo Credit: Stephanie Detjen Costabel*

# 24

*November 21, 2019*
*The worst day of my life.*

Alessia slept for the rest of the day once we got back from our appointment with Dr. Perez. She hadn't vomited again and hadn't had diarrhea, so I was hoping that what she had was just a virus and she was just tired from fighting it.

The next day was our IEP meeting at Hickory Grove Elementary School to discuss Alessia's goals at school. IEPs are Individualized Education Plans for special-needs children to help them best learn in the education system. She was still extremely lethargic and uncomfortable. I was glad when the meeting was over. Something was awfully wrong. She couldn't keep her eyes open. Her color was off. She was so pale. I had no idea what was wrong. I started wondering if it could be a shunt malfunction. She had all the classic signs: vomiting, lethargy, irritability. But she didn't have papilledema when they checked her optic nerves during the corneal transplant, so I was not for sure whether she was in shunt failure. I called Dr. Van Poppel's office and left a message for the nurse.

By 6 p.m. that night, I was extremely worried. Alessia had slept all day. She hadn't urinated since the morning. I paced from one side of my house to the other, wondering if I should take her to the ER. She had not thrown up since the night before—maybe I should just give it time? By 8 p.m., she finally woke up and started projectile vomiting.

I couldn't wait any longer. I had to take her in. Ronaldo put Alessia in her car seat, as I grabbed a backpack with clothes and her feeding supplies and headed to the Emergency Room. I glanced at Alessia through the rearview mirror every five minutes. She looked lifeless.

I pressed on the gas. *Please, God. It's the shunt. Shit. I know it is. Please, God.*

Tears started streaming down my cheeks. This was life threatening. Shivers went down my spine. This was serious. I knew it was.

I stormed into the ER and went straight to the front desk. Alessia started vomiting again as I walked in. "Please! She has a shunt. I think it's malfunctioning. Please! She needs to be seen right now!" I screamed.

The receptionist pulled up Alessia's chart and immediately sent us back to the ER rooms.

The ER was full that night. There wasn't a room available, so they had us wait in the hallway. One of the ER nurses put a pulse oximeter sensor on Alessia's toe to monitor her stats, while we waited for a room to become available.

"We're here waiting in the hallway," I said to Ronaldo over the phone. "I bet you anything it's the shunt. She started throwing up again as soon as we got here." I was sitting on the hospital bed in the hallway, holding Alessia who was fast asleep again. "The good thing is that they are going to go ahead and order a shunt series CT scan and a rapid sequence MRI, but I'm almost positive it's the shunt. I doubt they'll be able to do any surgery right now though, because she has to be NPO for at least six hours." NPO means she must have nothing to eat or drink. The last time I'd fed her was just an hour or two ago.

Suddenly Alessia started shaking and jerking her arms and legs. I dropped my phone. "Oh my God!" I screamed. "Help! She's having a seizure!!!"

I got up from the bed and ran to the nurse station carrying Alessia's jerking body.

"Help! Oh my God! She's never had a seizure before. PLEASE HELP!" I let out a sobbing cry. I was shaking so badly I couldn't even hold Alessia and handed her over to the nurse.

"I need help here!" the nurse called as she cleared one of the ER rooms and put Alessia on her side on the hospital bed and started stroking her back fast.

Within thirty seconds, there was a whole team of people in the room. One nurse was trying to start an IV, while the other nurse was trying to suction out her throat from her own secretions. I saw blood pouring out of her nose. I backed away and tried to catch my breath as I sobbed. "What's going on? PLEASE! It's her shunt. I know it is. She's in shunt failure. We need to get a CT scan right now!" I could barely breathe.

The nurse placed two IVs in her tiny little arms. They withdrew blood from one IV and administered Ativan through the other IV to control her seizure.

The ER doctor called down to the MRI room. "We need an emergent CT scan and rapid sequence MRI for a child with suspected shunt failure," I heard her say.

Alessia's nose continued bleeding from the suction machine being shoved down her nostrils to clear her airway from her secretions. I felt like I was going to vomit. She looked pale, lifeless, and was desaturating her oxygen levels to the 60s. They secured an oxygen cannula on her nose and slowly, her stats came up.

"We're going to wheel her down to MRI right now," the ER doctor said to me as she nodded at the nurse. "Take the Ativan just in case she seizes again," she told the nurse.

I looked to the floor and my phone was laying there. Ronaldo had not hung up. He was hearing the whole chaotic scene unfold.

I grabbed my phone. "Oh my God! Did you hear what just happened?" I asked. My voice was shaking. I was pacing back and forth from one side of the room to the other.

Ronaldo was crying. "Just please call me once they do the MRI."

I held Alessia's hand while the nurse wheeled her down to the CT scan room. She was asleep, but so pale, and every once in a while, her body would tremble. "Is that normal?" I kept asking the nurse.

"Her stats are normal," she replied as she glanced at the monitor.

I crawled in with her into the CT scanner. She was completely asleep and still. *God, please let her survive.*

Watching her have a grand mal seizure had scared the living shit out of me.

We were in the scanner for about five minutes while they took the images of her brain. "It will all be over soon, I promise," I whispered into her ear. She hadn't woken up since the seizure.

"Okay, now we have to go down to MRI," the nurse said as she wheeled Alessia down the hall.

"My sweet Alessia, I am so sorry," I said as I caressed her face. She was so pale.

Her body started shaking again. I glanced at the monitor. She was desaturating. My heart started pounding as I watched the numbers of her oxygen levels decline . . . 79, 75, 60, 50, 40 . . .

"I need back-up in MRI!" the nurse called on her phone.

"Why is she shaking? Oh my God! She is desaturating! She's in the 40s!" I was panicking. I was shaking like crazy.

"I am going to give her another dose of Ativan. She is having another seizure. Don't worry. Worst case scenario, if she codes, I will perform CPR," the nurse said.

*CPR? Please, God. No.*

I was dizzy and leaned on the wall of the hallway to catch my balance and not faint.

"Let's take her upstairs to stabilize her," the ER doctor said as soon as she came down to MRI. "We will abort the MRI until she's stable," she told the MRI technician as she wheeled Alessia back to the ER.

*This can't be happening.*

"Let's get her on a high-flow CPAP with oxygen," the ER doctor told the nurse once we were back in the ER room.

The neurosurgery resident on call was waiting for me when we came back to the ER.

"I reviewed her results from the CT scans she just had, and it doesn't appear to me that this is a shunt issue. Her ventricles are normal. There is no evidence of shunt malfunction." He pressed on the shunt reservoir to check the flow. Usually if there is a shunt malfunction the shunt reservoir would feel hard and not pump back up when he pressed on it. Alessia's reservoir was not hard and filled back up with fluid when he pressed on it.

"Well then what the hell is it?" I asked. "She has had shunt failure in the past and the scans have always been normal. We can't just go by a scan. I mean, look at her!" I glanced over to Alessia.

"I just pressed on her shunt reservoir, and it filled normally. This isn't the shunt," he assured me.

"Platelets are 14, Hemoglobin 5.7," the ER doctor said as she stormed into the room with the blood test results in her hands. The monitors started alarming. Alessia was desaturating her oxygen levels again.

The ER doctor looked at me and furrowed her eyebrows. "We have contacted the Pediatric ICU. She needs to be admitted. The PICU doctor is heading over here now to talk to you."

Tears were streaming down my face. I couldn't understand any of it. What the hell was going on? If it wasn't the shunt, then what was it?

I called my mom. "Ma, you need to come to Levine. Alessia is getting admitted to the PICU. She's had a grand mal seizure." I choked on my sobs.

My mother had just arrived home from her Spain vacation that same day.

"I'm heading over there now," she said.

Nobody could explain to me with certainty what was going on because nobody really knew. She was extremely anemic, platelets dangerously low. Everything pointed to something in her blood.

My mother arrived at the same time the PICU doctor came. I hugged her and sobbed. I was so scared. Not even my mother's hugs could calm me down.

"Hi, I am Dr. Kole from PICU." I heard the doctor's voice in the background. I looked over my shoulder.

"Can you explain to me what's going on?" I asked. I was choking on my sobs.

"Alessia is dangerously hemolytic. There is some kind of blood disorder going on that we still do not know. She needs to have a platelet transfusion right now. I do want to let you know that if she cannot maintain her oxygen saturations at a healthy number, we will have to intubate her."

My eyes widened. No. The thought of intubating her made shivers go down my spine. I knew she was a difficult airway intubation.

She was wheeled up to PICU. They were manually injecting platelets into her IV. I thanked God for blood donors.

At around 1:15 a.m. they made the call to intubate. She was not protecting her airway and kept desaturating dangerously low. We were losing her.

The PICU team spent two hours trying to intubate her. I paced from one side of the PICU hallway to the other, sobbing. My mother was sobbing too but trying to maintain herself for my sake. My stomach was feeling the effects of the anxiety and panic, and I vomited and had diarrhea while I waited.

I walked in front of her room constantly . . . trying to get a glimpse of what was happening. I couldn't see Alessia. There were too many people in her room. All I could see was the ER doctor making phone calls. They couldn't intubate her. Her airway was too difficult.

Finally, around 4 a.m., the anesthesia team arrived and successfully intubated her.

She was in a medically induced coma, but she was stable. She had not died, but I felt my soul die that night.

The fear of losing your child is incomparable to any other fear. She was in kidney failure and after they were done with her that night, I could hardly recognize my child.

Alessia lay lifelessly on the hospital bed with a breathing tube down her throat. She had IVs all over both her arms. I looked at her groin and gasped. A tube the size of a water hose was connected through a catheter to the left of her groin. It was pulling blood out of her body and into a dialysis machine. To the right of her groin was another tube the size of a water hose, pumping healthy, filtered blood back into her body.

Her head was wrapped with white gauze protecting the EEG sensors. They were doing an EEG study to see if she was still having seizures. She was swollen all over. I assumed it was from all the steroids they'd given her. The beeping sounds of the twenty machines all around her made chills go down my spine. I sat on the couch next to the hospital bed and covered my face with my hands.

"We think it might be Thrombotic Thrombocytopenic Purpura or Atypical Hemolytic Uremic Syndrome," Dr. Kole said as he wrote on the dry-erase board: "TTP or AHUS."

I raised my head and turned my attention towards him.

"TTP is a blood disorder in which platelet clumps form in small blood vessels. This leads to a low platelet count. It is caused by problems with an enzyme that is involved in blood clotting. This enzyme is called ADAMTS13. Absence of this enzyme results in platelet clumping. Platelets are a part of the blood that aids in blood clotting."

He continued, "As the platelets clump together, fewer platelets are available in the blood in other parts of the body to help with clotting. This can lead to bleeding under the skin and can lead to organ failure. We have sent her blood to see if this enzyme is present. If it is present, we can rule out TTP and concentrate on HUS, which can be Atypical." He paused to clear his throat.

"HUS is a condition that affects the blood and blood vessels. It results in the destruction of blood platelets, a low red blood cell count and kidney failure due to damage to the very small blood vessels of the kidneys.

"HUS usually happens after a severe bowel infection with certain toxic strains of the bacteria E. coli. Has she had severe diarrhea recently?" Dr. Kole asked.

"She has had diarrhea, but not severe. Can we send her blood to see if she was infected with E. coli?" I asked.

"Yes. We already have. We will have the results in a couple of hours." He furrowed his eyebrows. "If the E. Coli detection test comes back negative, then we can assume she has Atypical Hemolytic Uremic Syndrome, which is genetic. We would have to send her blood to the University of Iowa to see if there are genes that are related to AHUS. Either way, Nephrology has been called and they will be here in a couple of hours to talk to you about this. Right now, we just have to wait until all the lab results come back." He put his hand on my shoulder. "I'm so sorry this is happening."

"Does the corneal transplant have anything to do with this? It seems too coincidental for the timing."

"We have been in contact with the Duke Eye Center, and they are researching if corneal transplants have anything to do with any of these blood disorders since it is extremely rare. We should hear from them soon." He got up from the couch.

"Is she going to die?" I asked. My voice trembled and I let out a sob.

"I would be surprised if she were to die right now. She is intubated. The ventilator is breathing for her. We just have to wait and hope she heads towards the right direction and recovers." He left the room.

It was 5 a.m. and I just sat there on the couch, looking at my daughter. At some point, I passed out from exhaustion. I was awakened a couple hours later to the sound of my husband's sobs.

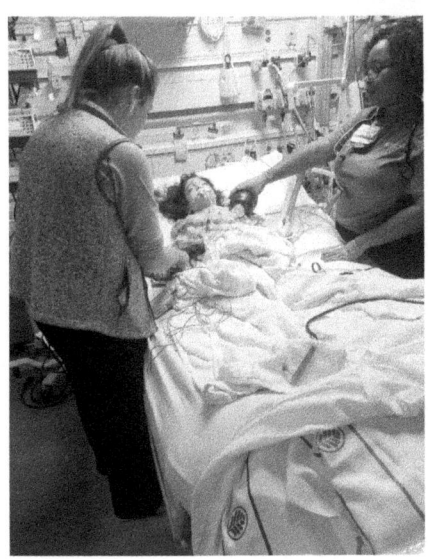 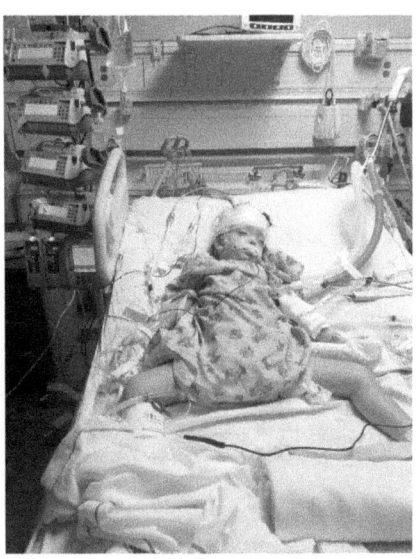

*Worst day of my life,*
*November 21, 2019*
*Photo Credit: Stephanie Detjen Costabel*

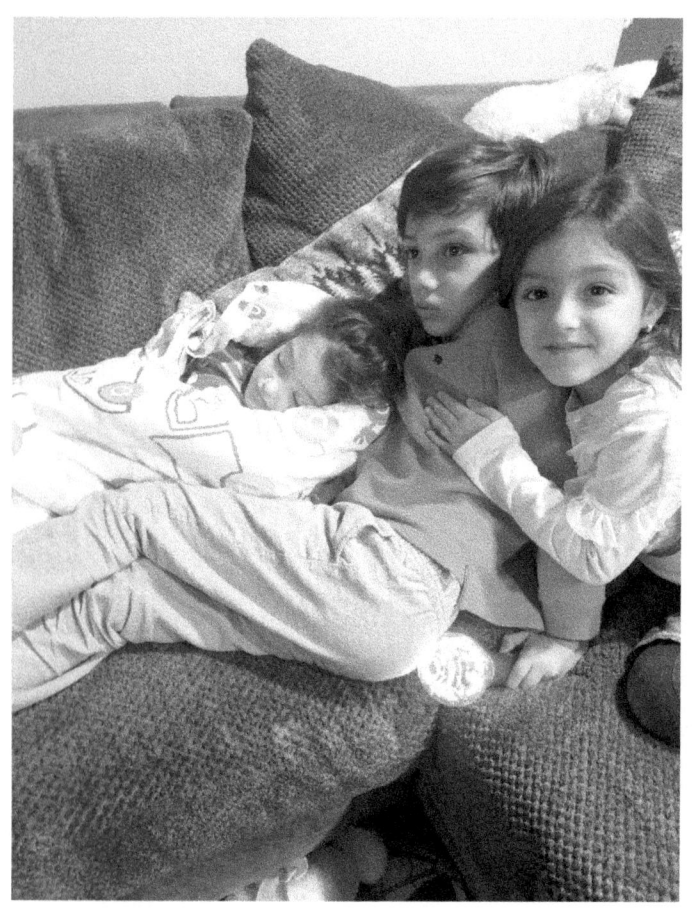

*Thiago and Sophia taking care of Alessia
right before taking her to the ER.
Photo Credit: Stephanie Detjen Costabel*

## 25

I looked up and saw Ronaldo, face in his hands, crying. He had come to bring me breakfast. He had never seen Alessia like this. He couldn't hold back the desperation he felt. He was supposed to be the protector. But we could not protect her right now, only the medical professionals could protect her and God . . . if he existed.

I had never seen him cry the way he cried that day. I walked over to him and put my arms around his shoulders, crying quietly along with him. Two parents . . . watching their child, so fragile and ill. The connection we shared at that moment was intense. But neither one of us could protect each other, and we could not protect Alessia. We had to rely on the doctors and medicine. We couldn't even pray. We were both so angry at God that we had no energy left to beg. We only hoped for the best and put our trust in the PICU doctor's medical expertise.

It was 10 a.m. before I went home. Ronaldo stayed with Alessia in the PICU so I could go home and rest a little bit from the worst night of my life. Thankfully, the kids were at school and didn't know anything of what had happened.

I got home and called Dr. Williams. It had been a few days since he had done her corneal transplant.

"I am so incredibly sorry, Stephanie, Levine called me last night and told me Alessia was dangerously ill." He paused and cleared his throat. "I cannot find anything in medical literature that could involve the corneal transplant to the blood disorder she developed."

"What about the Oxervate drops?" I asked as I paced around my kitchen island in circles. "These eye drops are extremely new. It has only been recently FDA approved. Aren't these drugs made in E. coli?"

"I have contacted Dompe Pharmaceuticals to get more information regarding these eye drops, but the blood disorder that your daughter has has not been reported as a side effect from using Oxervate."

"Well, I am definitely stopping the drops just in case."

"I completely understand. I probably would too. I'm going to keep researching and I will call you if I find anything."

"Thank you, Dr. Williams."

I sat on my couch trying to process everything that had just happened the night before.

Why my daughter? No child should ever have to go through this. *God! If you're up there, please . . . please don't let her die!* I kneeled on the floor and begged as I sobbed. I was terrified.

At some point I fell asleep and was awakened four hours later by the sound of my ringtone. It was Ronaldo.

"How is she?" I asked, my heart racing.

"Stable for now. Nephrology is coming to talk to us in a few minutes."

"Heading over there now." I hung up the phone, took a quick shower, and headed to Levine.

Before I entered Alessia's room, I took a deep breath to prepare myself. I walked in and took a quick look at Alessia—she was so swollen. Ronaldo was on the couch, his eyes red and puffy from crying. The nurse was removing the EEG sensors from her head.

An older doctor I had never seen before was standing by her bedside.

"Hi, Mom, I'm Dr. Kirby, I'm with Nephrology." She looked at me and smiled. "I was just about to give your husband an update." I'd arrived just at the right time. I sat on the couch next to Ronaldo and gave Dr. Kirby my undivided attention.

"We received the results of the Adams TS3 blood test. The enzyme is present in her blood so we can rule out TTP. We suspect she has Atypical Hemolytic Uremic Syndrome."

"Do we have the results of the E. coli test?" I interrupted.

She glanced over to the nurse. "I think we do. Can you check on that for me, please?" she asked the nurse.

The nurse clicked on the lab results on her computer. "It came back negative."

"With Hemolytic Uremic Syndrome, we would see severe, bloody diarrhea and she has not had that, correct?" she asked us.

"She has had bouts of diarrhea here and there for the past week, but it has not been bloody," I said. I glanced at Alessia's groin. My sweet girl. Tubes were coming out all over her body. She looked so lifeless.

"So, AHUS, which is Atypical Hemolytic Uremic Syndrome, is treated with Solaris, which is an IV immunosuppressant therapy, a class of chemotherapy that helps manage this blood disorder. At some point, we will have to place a port-a-cath in her chest for future IV infusions."

"Future IV infusions?! What do you mean?!"

Dr. Kirby frowned. "Unfortunately, this is long-term care. She will need to have these infusions every two weeks . . . for life."

I swallowed hard as I covered my face with my hands and let out a cry. "Are you serious?" I asked. I was in shock. I felt Ronaldo hold my hand.

"So, with AHUS, a part of the immune system called the complement system becomes active when it shouldn't be. Solaris contains a humanized antibody that binds to the last protein in the complement pathway, preventing it from completing the activation of the immune response." She sighed, swallowed, and continued. "In most cases, AHUS is genetic. So, we are going to send her blood to the University of Iowa, who does the genetic testing, to see if she has the gene that causes AHUS. The problem is that it does take a few months to get the results back."

"So, it is safe to say we don't know exactly if she has AHUS until we get the genetic panel back, correct?" I asked.

"We are almost certain she does have AHUS, but yes. It will be confirmed with the results of her genetic testing." Dr. Kirby handed me a pamphlet with information on AHUS and Solaris. "We started her with the first round of Solaris a couple of hours ago and we will do a second round in three days."

"Can we wait until we have the results of the genetic testing before putting a port-a-cath in her chest?" I asked as I put the pamphlet down on the couch.

"Absolutely. We don't have to place the port-a-cath right now. We don't have to do it in this hospital stay, but given how sick she is, she needs to continue on Solaris for a few months. It's given in the Infusion Center up on the fifth floor. They will have to put an IV in every time she goes. It takes roughly two hours to administer the drug, and it's given every two weeks."

I sighed and nodded.

As Dr. Kirby was heading out, Dr. Kole was walking in. "Did you get any sleep?" he asked us.

I yawned. "A little, yes."

"So, um, with her kidney failure, her blood pressure. She has high blood pressure that we are managing with blood pressure medication. Hopefully, as her kidneys recover, we can wean her down the blood pressure meds. She will need to be on blood pressure medicine for a few months until her blood pressure stabilizes." He scratched the side of his well-kept beard.

I nodded as I tried to focus on what he was telling me. There was a lot to process, and we were getting hit with bad news after bad news.

"Do you happen to have any good news?" I asked and immediately regretted my question. She was alive.

"There is, actually." He smiled. "Her EEG showed she has not had any seizures since she was admitted to the ER. So thankfully we can rule out epilepsy."

Thank God.

"How long will she be intubated?" I asked.

"Most likely for several days. She is not close to extubation anytime soon."

He left us a little while later.

I wanted my daughter back. Her wild, hyper, stubborn personality. I wanted to see her awake, running through the hallways. I wanted to see her yanking her IVs out of her arms like she always did. I wanted to see her destroying my plants and taking off her shoes. Seeing her this way—lying lifelessly on the bed with a tube down her throat, in a medically induced coma, broke my heart into a million pieces.

At least she was alive. She could have died. We could have lost her last night. A pain no mother should ever have to feel.

"She is completely sedated, paralyzed with loads of pain medications. She is not feeling a thing, I promise," the night shift nurse said to me.

It was comforting to know she wasn't feeling pain. With all the IVs and tubes running out of her body, I was glad she was getting high doses of narcotics. We had made it through day number two, and I was so incredibly relieved.

## 26

After seven long days in a medically induced coma, Alessia was finally extubated.

I was amazed at the power of medicine. Her kidneys had recovered. Her platelets were coming back to normal. Her swelling had gone down. Her labs were normalizing. We were being moved down to Progressive Care. Discharge was closer and closer.

I thought when they extubated Alessia, she would immediately sit up and cry for me to hold her. I thought she would be back to her normal self, but I was wrong.

Alessia had bitten her tongue when she had her grand mal seizure in the ER. It was swollen, protruding from her mouth, and she was unable to put her tongue back into her mouth. She was extremely debilitated, and her muscles deconditioned. She couldn't move. She was lying there, unable to cry, unable to move, and just stared at the ceiling. I was heartbroken all over again. She looked so extremely sad. I hated that she had to go through this, but at least she was alive, I kept reminding myself.

Once she was stable enough and a room became available in Progressive Care we were wheeled over. As I walked the hallways of the PICU, memories flooded my mind of the night we almost lost her. I sighed as a tear ran down my cheek. *Thank God we are out of this place.*

Progressive Care had a much more relaxing feel to it. One nurse was usually assigned to two or three patients, as opposed to PICU who had one nurse assigned to each patient since they were so ill. Patients in the Progressive Care were stable. They were recovering. They were not in immediate life-threatening danger. It was so much more peaceful than the PICU.

I was warned she was going to be deconditioned since she was intubated for so long and it would take time for her to come to baseline. I had to have patience. She would be back to her usual self in no time, I kept assuring myself.

I brought in her favorite beads and her favorite toys. I flooded her room with balloons, anything that would motivate her to move and make her happy. But she barely moved for the first two days after she was extubated. I was beginning to lose hope.

"I'm just scared she will never be back to her normal self!" I cried as I talked to Mika on the phone. "They are going to do another EEG tonight because they feel like she's having partial seizures. She barely opens her eyes. Her team of specialists wants to order another MRI, just to make sure there wasn't residual damage to the brain the night she was admitted to the ER." I held my breath trying to control my cries. "But they said it can also be withdrawals from all the narcotics she was on while she was in the PICU."

"Well," Mika said, "just think, she was in a medically induced coma for eight days, so of course she will be deconditioned. I mean, it could very well be withdrawals. Give it time."

Mika was by my side every step of the way, guiding me and helping me think rationally. The what ifs were what was killing me. What if she never walks again? What if she did have damage to the brain and she never goes back to her usual self? I just wanted my daughter back.

"Well, the good news is she didn't have any seizures during the EEG," the neurologist told me the following day. "She did show abnormal focal activity that could lead to a seizure, but I think putting her on a low dose of Keppra will prevent a seizure from developing."

I let out a sigh of relief.

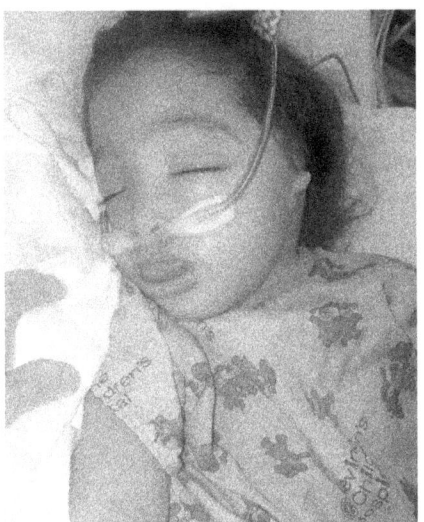 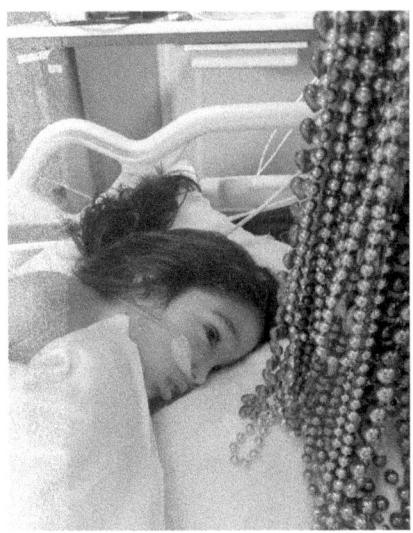

*Alessia after extubation, December 2019*
*Photo Credit: Stephanie Detjen Costabel*

## 27

Thiago and Sophia were asking about their sister. I had tried to keep it short and not go into details about all that had happened to her, but they were beginning to sense something was not right. They hadn't seen their sister in thirteen days.

I decided to take them to visit Alessia. Alessia was still not walking and extremely deconditioned, but she was starting to move around more, so she was heading in the right direction. I was extremely relieved to find out the MRI revealed her brain had not had any residual damage.

"Oh my God, what happened to her?" Thiago cried as he put his face in his hands. "I want my sister back! Why is her tongue like that? Why isn't she walking? Why is she so sad?" he asked in between sobs.

I tried to hold back my tears.

"She will be back in no time, baby. She just was very, very sick and she isn't feeling well. But she is still the same Alessia." I looked over to Sophia. She was too young to really understand.

"No, she's not!" he yelled at me. "How is she the same? Do you not see how her tongue is?" He was so angry.

I looked at her blistered, swollen, protruding tongue.

"It's going to get better, baby. I promise."

I swallowed hard as I looked the other way so he wouldn't see my tears.

Something unexplainably magical happened with Alessia that night. I wasn't sure if it was her brother and sister visiting, or my mom singing to her, but something in her brain clicked and she suddenly sat up from her bed. She looked around and started climbing off the bed! I smiled from ear to ear and immediately went to her bedside. She wanted to walk! And even better, she went to go sit on the toilet and actually peed! Her kidneys were working!

I called the nurse so we could disconnect her from her IVs for a little bit so she could walk around.

She walked independently all down the Progressive Care hallways, stopping and exploring the different textures of the walls. She continued to be intrigued by the strangest things. But the best news was my girl was coming back. She was showing us a glimpse of her personality we thought we'd lost.

Tears of joy ran down my cheeks. Alessia was still the same Alessia, and I couldn't have felt happier.

After sixteen long, nerve-wracking days in the hospital, Alessia was discharged.

I wheeled the cart full of balloons, toys, and all our bags through the front doors of Levine Children's Hospital, a tear of relief rolling down my cheek. Ronaldo was right behind me, carrying Alessia. She marveled at the shiny Christmas ornaments on the huge Christmas tree standing in the lobby of the hospital. I looked back and smiled. *Thank you, Levine, for saving my daughter's life.*

It took two months for Alessia to be able to put her tongue back into her mouth. It would blister, ooze pus, and every time I tried to clean it, she would bite on it all over again and it would swell up again. She was petrified of anything going close to her mouth. My poor daughter had PTSD after all she had been through.

The biweekly Solaris infusions were terrible. They could never find a good vein, so they always had to poke her more than once to place an IV in, and then she would scream and cry the whole infusion trying to yank her IV out. But I preferred her like this—a fighter—than how she had been when she was in coma. But it still hurt my soul to see her in pain.

The fact that she couldn't talk or hear made it so much worse. I hated I couldn't explain to her that the infusions were for her own good.

The corneal transplant was stable, but it had rejected, so her cornea slowly began to cloud up and she lost most of her central vision in that eye. But we still had the right eye, which was intact, thankfully.

By March of 2020, she had developed a hernia that needed surgical repair. One more surgery to add to her list of medical interventions.

But once again, I was amazed by how quickly she bounced right back after her surgery. She was fearless, determined, and extremely strong.

After her hernia repair surgery, she refused to wear diapers or shorts or anything that went over her waistline. Not even underwear. We had a lot of accidents. I was warned it was going to be hard to potty train her, but eventually she got it. I was amazed at how incredibly brilliant she was. With no hearing and only one eye with good vision, she somewhat understood what was going on in her environment. She was amused at watching me clean her poop and pee from the floor. There was a stage in her potty training where she would go and sit on the toilet but go right on the edge, so all the pee would land on the floor. She would poop on the carpet or on the floor and play with her poop. She was so mischievous. It is called fecal smearing and is quite common with kids who have cognitive disabilities. I knew she knew it was wrong because every time she did it, she would laugh.

There were times where I cleaned poop and pee from the floor every single day. I invested in a good carpet cleaner, and I was washing my carpet on a daily basis. It bothered me, but I tried to never complain. I preferred her like this than in coma like she had been a few months before.

She enjoyed the hell out of our Make-A-Wish hydrotherapy tub that whole summer of 2020. Covid-19 didn't really bother us. We lived in our own little world in our backyard. I was incredibly grateful my daughter was alive and striving.

The AHUS hospitalization changed me. I was never the same. We had been so close to losing her that I learned to appreciate life more. I let her do whatever she wanted. I was determined to make her as happy as possible. She would be in the jacuzzi completely naked every single minute of the day. She loved it. Water had always been her favorite thing in the whole wide world. And she adored being naked. She didn't care who was present. She had a free spirit and would be naked in front of the president of the United States and not care. I loved to see her so wild and alive and back to her stubborn personality. It was hard work on my end, but that was fine. All I wanted was for her to have fun and be happy. And if her happiness was nudity, then nude she would be.

We got the results of the genetic testing from the University of Iowa, and they couldn't find any gene in Alessia's blood that was related to AHUS, so by May of 2020 we decided to stop the biweekly Solaris infusions. She did extremely well, and Nephrology just monitored her labs periodically to make sure her platelets were normal, and her kidney function maintained itself.

We did a yearly checkup of her Chiari, and everything was stable. Her Chiari hadn't really changed, and Cranio Cervical Instability was not present. The fusion surgery was being put on hold. I didn't want to even think of a fusion surgery after all she had been through. I often wonder if I should just never do a fusion and let her enjoy her life, regardless of how many years she lives. I had seen her so ill and so close to death that I didn't want to put her through anymore suffering.

School was placed on hold due to the Covid pandemic. We had tried Zoom with Alessia, but it wasn't really going anywhere, so I opted out of school for her. Everything was going so well, it scared me. It was as if I was just waiting for something bad to happen. I had severe PTSD. I started going to therapy and started taking antidepressants. Being a parent of a child so medically complex can make you feel like you are dying. You try so incredibly hard to give your child the best quality of life possible. You want them to not hurt. You want to have a conversation with them like a normal child. You want, with all the power in your soul, for them to understand how incredibly loved they are and how sorry you are that they have a life with so many obstacles. You fear. You are always in fear that they will die. And you will never accept it. All these thoughts mess with your brain . . . and you become depressed, overly anxious, and extremely sentimental.

Exactly one year after the worst day of my life, Alessia managed to perforate her only good eye, her right eye. Her addiction to eye poking had come back in the fall, and history repeated itself with a non-healing ulcer. This time it was in the only eye she had good vision in. We tried everything. She had sedated eye exams with Dr. Perez at the Duke Eye Center on a weekly basis. We tried Amniotic Membrane Transplants, Autologous Serum Tears, patching, contact bandages. Everything. But her eye eventually perforated, and she ended up having an emergency corneal transplant . . . that with time . . . also rejected.

I was devastated. It was the only sense she had left that connected her to the world. She was now legally blind in both eyes and profoundly deaf.

I spent night and day trying to research anything that would improve her vision. She could see some light and see shadows, but her corneas were opaque, white from the corneal transplant rejections. Her visual acuity was severely impacted, as well as her depth perception. She couldn't see one foot away from her.

But she was incredibly adaptable, amazing us all. She learned to use her touch and the little vision she had to find whatever it was she wanted. When she was hungry, she would find her feeding tube syringe and hand it to me. When she wanted to go outside, she would feel for my hand and take me to the doorknob. When she was thirsty, she would bring me a bottle of water. When she was tired, she would take me to her bed so I could tuck her in. When she needed to go to the bathroom, she would take me to the bathroom doorknob. She's ridiculously intelligent.

I often wonder how high her IQ really is, being able to somewhat communicate her needs with all the disabilities she has.

Researching night and day, I came across a glimpse of hope in recovering her vision: Corneal Neurotization. A novel procedure performed to treat corneal anesthesia.

Dr. Leyngold at the Duke Eye Center had invented a minimally invasive corneal neurotization technique to achieve successful restoration of corneal sensibility, health, and improved vision.

It was extremely new, though, and it wasn't guaranteed it was going to work on Alessia. Duke Eye Center hadn't discussed it to me previously because it was indeed a novel procedure.

It could take several months before she recovered sensation to her cornea and even then, it wasn't certain it would work given her trigeminal nerve anatomy. But there wasn't much left to lose: she was already severely visually impaired. If we had a chance to restore some vision in at least one of her eyes, then I was going to do it.

"Six months," Dr. Leyngold said to me. "It will probably be a fifty-fifty chance it will work. We will know for sure in approximately six months. We can expect for her to stop poking at her cornea because she will feel the pain, and hopefully this will prevent future corneal ulcerations."

"If this works," I asked, "will she be able to have a repeat corneal transplant in the future and hopefully maintain a clear cornea?"

"Absolutely," he replied.

I debated on doing this surgery for months. Her eye poking continued. I had to at least try before she poked the rest of her eyes out. I took the jump. And on May 6, 2021, Alessia went into her eighteenth surgery.

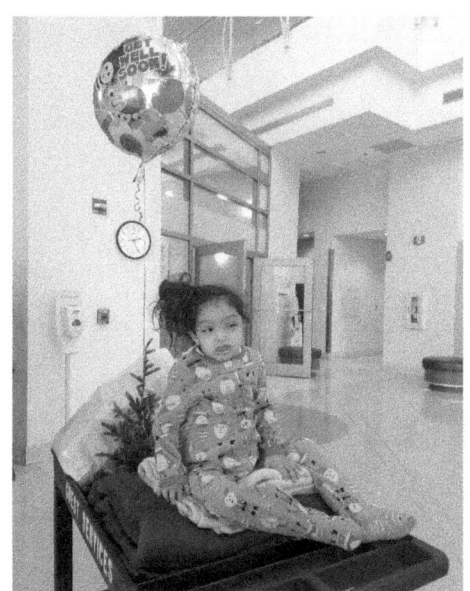
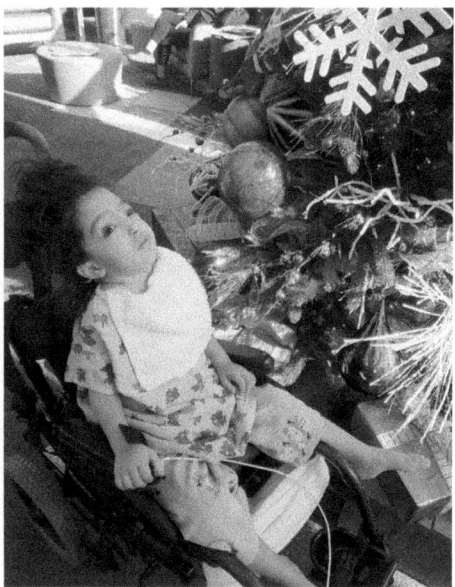

*Alessia on her discharge date, December 2019*
*Photo Credit: Stephanie Detjen Costabel*

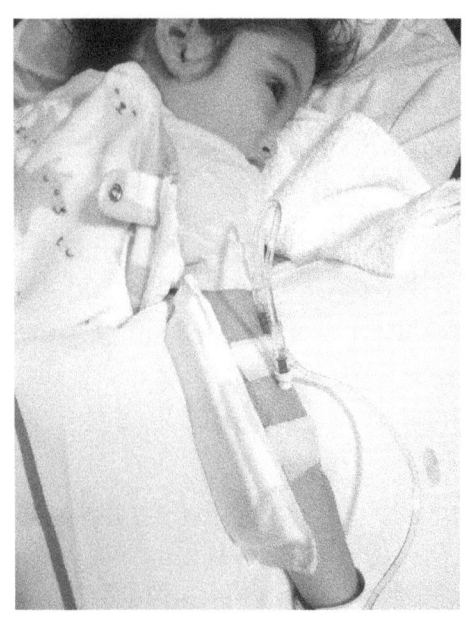
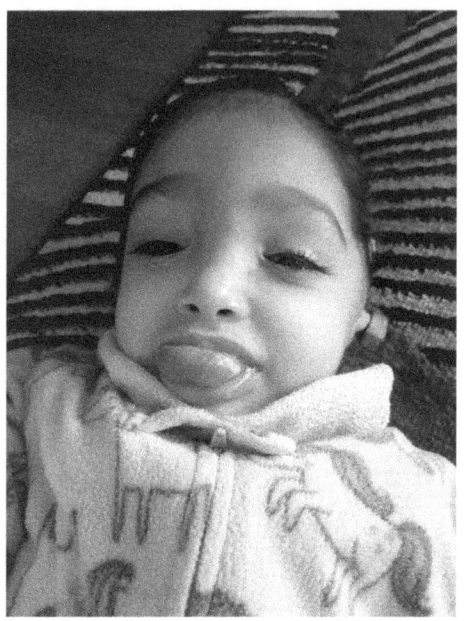

*Alessia at her infusion, 2020*
*Photo Credit: Stephanie Detjen Costabel*

*Alessia's protruding tongue, 2020*
*Photo Credit: Stephanie Detjen Costabel*

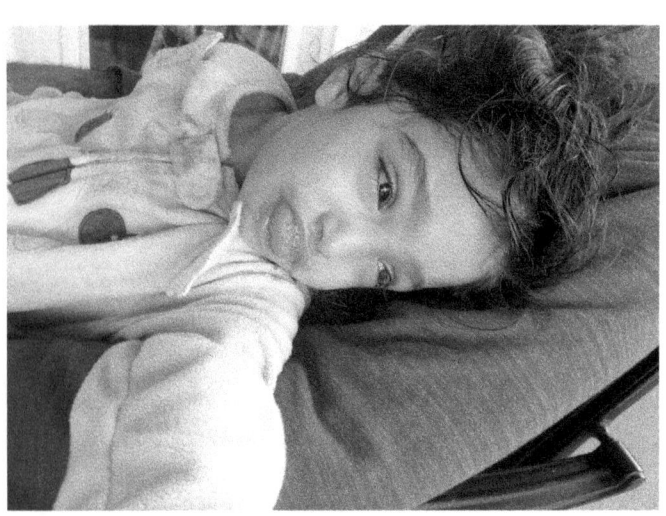

*Alessia biting her tongue, 2020*
*Photo Credit: Stephanie Detjen Costabel*

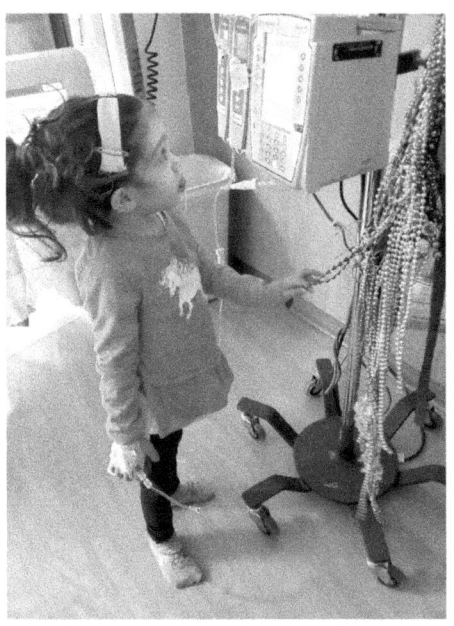

*Alessia at the infusion center, 2020*
*Photo Credit: Stephanie Detjen Costabel*

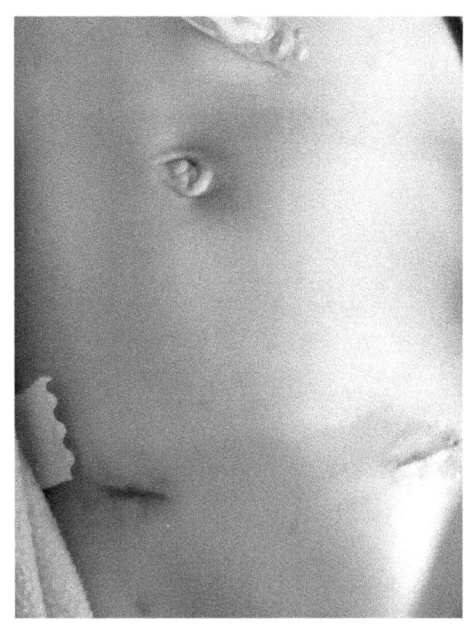

*Alessia's hernia repair surgery scars*
*Photo Credit: Stephanie Detjen Costabel*

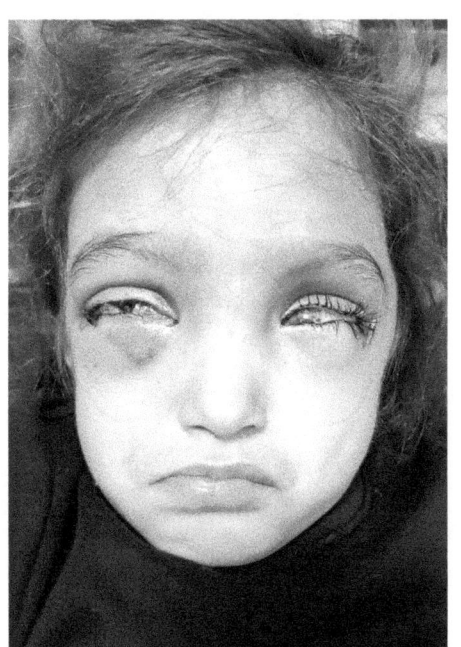

*Alessia two days after the corneal*
*neurotization procedure*
*Photo Credit: Stephanie Detjen Costabel*

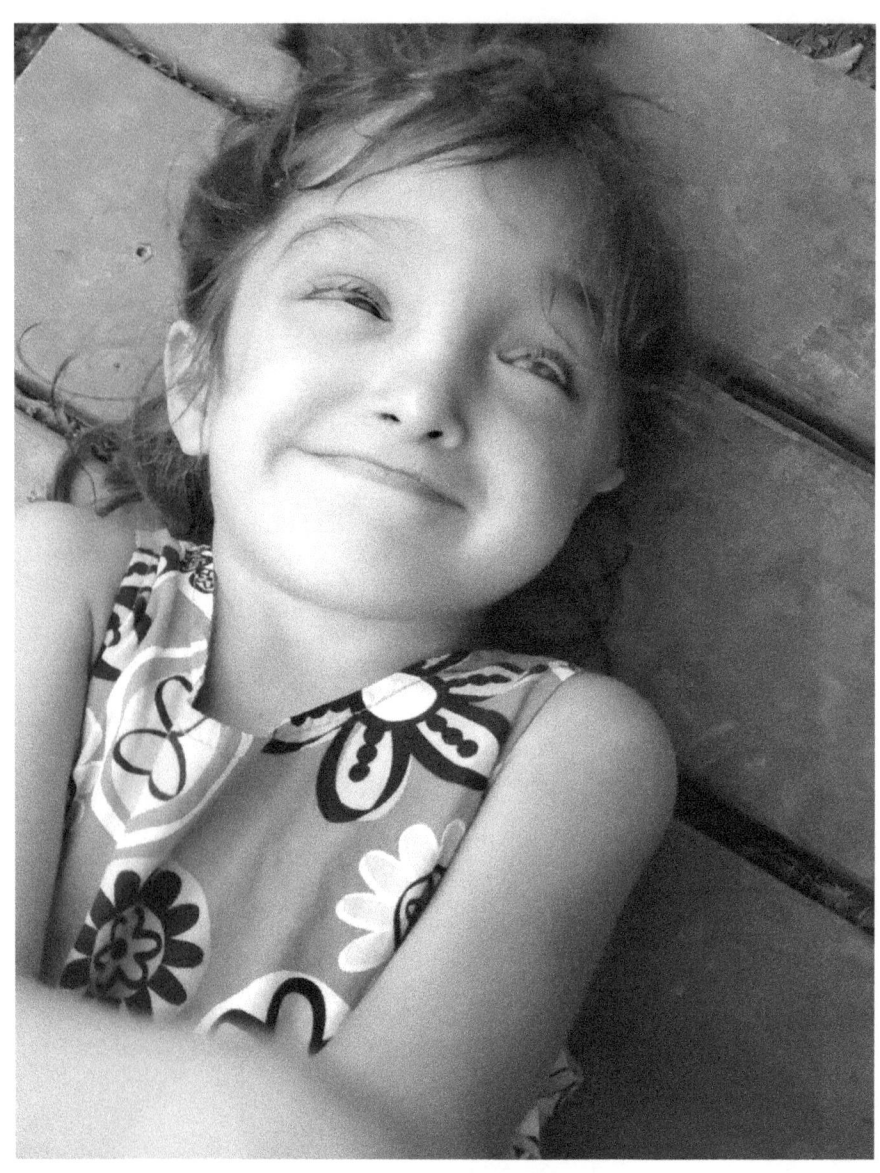

*Alessia on her 6th birthday*
*Photo Credit: Stephanie Detjen Costabel*

# Epilogue

Thankfully, after a few months, her corneal neurotization proved to be a success. Her vision improved. Dr. Leyngold also performed a partial tarsorrhaphy on the left eye that summer to help prevent future abrasions and maintain the cornea in optimal health. It's amazing how the eye has the potential to heal itself when it is partially shut. The tarsorrhaphy had dramatically improved the health of her eyes. With time, we noticed she wasn't picking at her eyes the way she used to.

I was grateful and hopeful.

As Alessia grows and gets older so does her physical strength. We now deal with other challenges. A six-year-old child who does not have speech to communicate their needs can be a dangerous situation. Alessia got into the habit of banging her head on the floor for every reason possible. If she was hungry, she head banged, if she was thirsty, she head banged, if she was tired . . . if she was bored . . . if she was in pain. Her forehead was always bruised and swollen, and at one point she had a deep forehead wound from so many head-banging episodes.

Watching your child self-injure themselves because they are uncomfortable and not able to communicate has been by far the biggest challenge I have ever faced in my journey with Alessia. It got to the point that we got psychiatry involved to try different medicines to help calm her down. She is strong. She punches us, kicks the floor, head bangs, and cries.

Have they worked?

Some do for a short period of time.

Alessia is a mystery impossible to solve. She metabolizes medicine differently than we do. One medicine will work one day but then you give her the same medicine the next day and it doesn't work. It is a guessing game with her. Are you hungry? Are you thirsty? Do you need to use the bathroom? Does your stomach hurt? Does your ear hurt? Do your eyes hurt? Does your head hurt? Are you bored? What could I possibly do to make you feel better? Questions I ask all day, every day.

She likes to be rocked, so I bought four different rocking chairs to place in different areas of our house. She still plays with beads, so I hung beads on every window seal.

The biggest obstacle is when she has some kind of pain that she cannot communicate, which is an everyday thing now. I start with gas drops if she passes a lot of smelly gas. If she hasn't had a bowel movement in a day or two, I give her a laxative or a suppository. Motrin has been the only medicine that has somewhat helped control her headaches. But even having her bowel movements, her stomach discomfort, and her head pain somewhat controlled she still manages to bang her head on the floor when she is feeling off. Not too long ago I took her to the dentist and found out her molars were coming in and it could be causing her discomfort.

Trips to the ER would only show moderate swelling on her forehead from head-banging but everything else always came back normal. It is also so bizarre how inconsistent her head-banging is nowadays. On a good day she might only head bang three or four times throughout the day, but on a bad day she head bangs over a hundred times a day. What all contributes to the bad days exactly? We still don't know.

## An Amazing Little Girl with Rhombencephalosynapsis

We gave ABA therapy another shot. Communication is what I desperately need from Alessia. I need to know what is discomforting her. Alessia's Developmental Pediatrician assured me that it was scientifically proven that ABA helped improve communication and decrease self-injurious behavior in children with autism. I had had an unpleasant experience with ABA three years ago, but I was also so desperate to help Alessia communicate and stop the constant self-injurious behavior that I decided to give it another chance. She has been in ABA for about a month now. I like the therapists working with her and they have been extremely understanding. They are taking it slowly.

The pain you feel when your child self-injures is intolerable. You feel helpless. Unable to understand. The not knowing is what drives me insane.

But we keep going . . . as a family. We are thankful she has made it to her sixth birthday. We are thankful she has not been hospitalized in over a year. We celebrate the victories. She is completely potty trained and has little to no accidents. Her vision has dramatically improved. We focus on the good days and try to forget the bad days. We explore options, ideas, anything that will help Alessia have less bad days.

We hope one day she will be able to live a life where she doesn't need to self-injure herself to communicate her needs with us. We hope one day she will be able to sit at the table with us and eat dinner. We hope to be able to have a conversation with her and talk about everyday things, like we do with Sophia and Thiago. We hope one day she can potentially live a pain-free life. Hope. The last thing we can ever lose. We hope. But until then, we have patience, we rejoice, and we continue living our lives with Our Amazing Little Girl with Rhombencephalosynapsis.

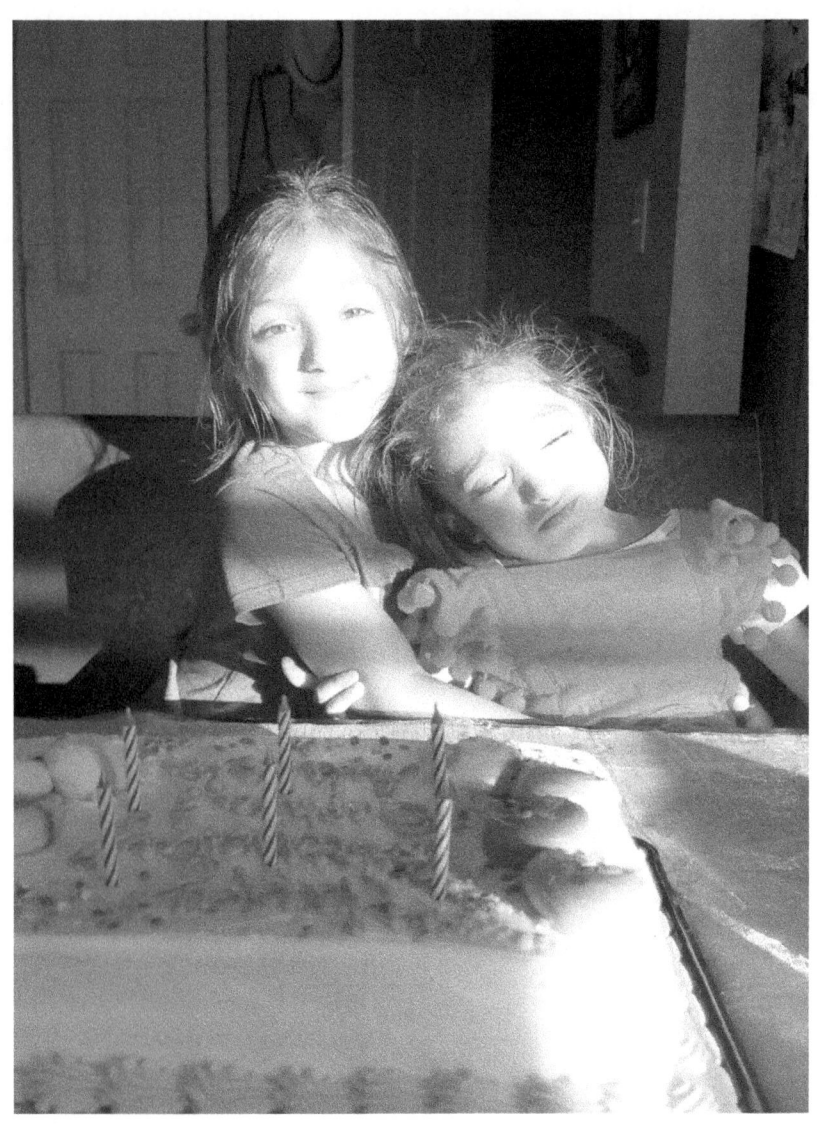

*Sophia and Alessia on their 6th birthday, April 2021*
*Photo Credit: Stephanie Detjen Costabel*

# Disclaimer

This memoir reflects my recollections of experiences and internal feelings over time. As the mother of Alessia Cruz, I shared our story the way our family lived and perceived it. I relied on past notes, medical history reports, communications with Alessia's team of specialists, and my own memory. Some names of people have been changed to protect their privacy. Some events and dialogues have been compressed. I have done my best to stick to the truth as much as possible. I regret any unintentional harm resulting from the publishing and marketing of *An Amazing Little Girl with Rhombencephalosynapsis*.